W9-AXF-130

AGAINST ALL ODDS

AGAINST ALL ODDS

Tom Helms

THOMAS Y. CROWELL PUBLISHERS

ESTABLISHED 1834   NEW YORK

FIRST EDITION

Designed by Sidney Feinberg

Library of Congress Cataloging in Publication Data

Helms, Tom.
  Against all odds.
    1. Tetraplegia—Biography. 2. Helms, Tom.
I. Title
RC406.T4H44   1978   362.4'3'0926 [B]   78–3302
ISBN 0–690–01763–4

78 79 80 81 82 10 9 8 7 6 5 4 3 2 1

FEB 4 81

For Nadine K.

For whom life was
an almost captured beauty

AGAINST ALL ODDS

PROLOGUE:

The Second Time

It wasn't the pain that woke me as much as it was a dull humming somewhere in the back of my head. There was the taste or smell of alcohol, I couldn't tell which, and I could almost hear my breath rasping through a smoke-dried chimney of a mouth. Hung over, I thought. And with the first stirrings of consciousness I could believe it, if only for a moment. I was hung over and last night the old nightmare had returned. I'd been having the same one for years, every time an arm or leg became entangled in the covers and movement was made difficult or stopped completely.

I lay with my eyes closed, drifting in a world not yet real, waiting for the gray to yield its shadowy secrets to the relentless, probing fingers of consciousness. I must have been drinking dynamite. I couldn't remember much about what happened. There had been men in white bolting a silver halo to the head of some errant angel. The poor son-of-a-bitch shouldn't have to be an angel if he didn't want to. I couldn't hold on to a thought. They kept rushing at me and melting away. I had fallen and couldn't get up. Things kept floating up out of the gray and disappearing back into it. Cory was fighting back the tears and trying not to show the fear. But the fear was there. I could see it in her eyes and in the tight set of her mouth. She began to fade. I wanted to say something, but the humming in my head was becoming a roar.

This isn't a hangover, I thought, as the gray began to yield to pinwheels and curves of bright flashing light. A hangover picks at you with quick jabs of pain and raises hell inside your skull. This was different. There was something sinister and familiar hiding beneath the roar. An old enemy that belonged in dreams.

I opened my eyes and squinted against the glare of a harsh white ceiling. The room began to spin and I felt sick. It was real! I couldn't clear my head or awaken fully, but it was real. I wasn't waking from a nightmare, I was waking into one.

"Oh God," I moaned, "please, no, not again."

I could speak! By God I could speak, and that meant no tube in my throat and if there was no tube in my throat then maybe it wasn't like before. All I had to do was move something, anything, an arm, a leg, a toe. That was it—a toe. I'd had enough practice. But if I tried and failed then it would all be true, none of it would have been a dream.

I closed my eyes and tried to feel as I had on a thousand other mornings. I wanted to hold on to it as long as I could, as long as there was any hope at all. It was early summer and the world was alive again after a long winter. There should be cotton candy puffs of white floating in a lazy blue sky. There should be the nervous chatter of squirrels chasing one another across a green expanse of lawn, the echoing of bird song, the drone of bees or some other winged insect humming me steadily awake. I should be glad to be awake, glad to be alive. But it wasn't any other morning. It was this morning and I was lying in a hospital, and there was the taste of medicine, and my head wouldn't clear, and the pain wouldn't stop.

I opened my eyes and closed them again when the ceiling

began to rock. It was hot. So hot that I couldn't breathe. I could only gasp and things were getting mixed up. There had been moments of consciousness during the night. Bits and pieces. But I didn't know. What was real and what wasn't, and now it was time to find out, only I didn't want to know.

"This is a gut check," Rick would say if he were here. "A goddamn ball-bustin' gut check. Let's see who's got 'em."

Well, I either had them or I didn't. I'd either move that toe or I wouldn't. I could feel myself slipping—gentle gray waves beginning to erode the edges of consciousness. I closed my eyes tight, trying to squeeze away the gray, and then I felt them. The tiny pin pricks of pain as my scalp tugged against the screws. The halo! Oh, God! It was real. It was all real.

I slipped back into dreams.

1

DREAMS had beckoned before. Gentle dreams that would steal away my life. It was four years earlier, and by fate or luck or those small details of chance that set the course of a man's life, I was conscious.

"Hold on. Hold on. Stay awake," they said.

Someone said it as they pulled me from the car in which I had hitched a ride. It was spring and I was on my way home from my first year of college. It was raining and the car skidded off the road and plunged down an embankment. It's funny what you think about at a time like that. As the car slid toward the embankment, all I could think of was that it was going to be a pain in the ass to lug my suitcase back up that wet bank. I could see myself slipping and sliding trying to get up that hill. My footing would fail and I would have to dig a knee and hand into the mud to keep from sliding all the way back down. I even got angry thinking about having to stand beside the road trying to hitch another ride in the rain with a muddy hand and two muddy knees.

There was the sound of glass breaking and metal tearing and then an eerie silence and the smell of fresh-plowed earth and gas. It takes a moment for orientation to come. It takes a moment for pain to come. I had never lain in the roof of a car with the back of the front seat slowly swaying above me before, so it took a moment to realize where I was and what everything was. I started to reach for the swaying seat and something exploded in my back. My vision faded and then came back. Pain, unspeakable pain, knifed into my back and shoulders. I tried to pull my shoulders back, to pinch my shoulder blades together and squeeze away the pain, but my shoulders wouldn't move. I tried to reach for the seat again. My arms wouldn't move. I had broken both shoulders. Jesus Christ, there goes the summer. Both arms in casts. The pain was clawing at my back, tearing and burning. Maybe I was lying on something sharp and it was being pressed deeper and deeper into me. I could roll off it if I used my legs. But I had to be careful. I had to be sure I rolled and didn't slide forward. If I pushed myself forward it would cut me open. I had to bring my legs up and push to one side. But my legs wouldn't move! They couldn't be broken. Broken legs hurt. I couldn't feel anything but the pain in my back. I couldn't really feel my legs. I'd feel them if they were broken. Maybe they were pinned under something. The suitcase? No, not the suitcase. I was too strong for that. The driver? The driver was lying on my legs. What's his name? What the hell's his name? He told me when he picked me up but I wasn't listening. I just wanted out of the rain. I never listen to people's names. I'm always thinking of what to say and I never hear their names.

Hey you, I said, only no sound came. My mouth moved and no sound came. I wasn't breathing. Oh, God, I wasn't breathing. I panicked. I started to scream and run, only I couldn't scream and I couldn't run. I was so scared I couldn't think. My mind flashed from one thought to another like a slide projector speeded up a thousand times. All kinds of thoughts about life and death and broken shoulders and casts and pain and bleeding to death and ragged metal stabbing into my back and not

5

breathing and what the guys would say when they heard old Tom had bought it and what a lousy place to die and what the hell's on my legs. I had to stop this. I had to think. Get hold of one thought and follow it through, then the next one, and pretty soon I'd figure a way out of this. I never had been in anything I couldn't get out of, and I could get out of this if I would only settle down and think.

If a person is bleeding from an artery and he's stopped breathing, what do you treat first? The bleeding or the breathing? The coach was always asking us that in health class and we were always missing it. "How long can you hold your breath, dumb ass?" he would yell. "Can you hold it a minute? Huh? One lousy minute? Well, I hope the hell you can because you can bleed to death in less than a minute."

I had to stop the bleeding first. Only I didn't know how. I wouldn't know how if I could get to it and I couldn't get to it. "Pressure, my young geniuses." Okay, you apply pressure. Stick a rag or something in there and press like hell. Only I haven't got a rag and my arms won't move and I can't get to my back.

Work on breathing. Forget about bleeding to death. You can't do anything about that, so forget it. But there was something wrong. If I wasn't breathing, why wasn't I getting dizzy? Why didn't my lungs feel as if they were going to explode the way they do when you've been under water too long and can't find the surface? I strained to feel with my body, to hear with my body. My chest wasn't moving. I wasn't breathing. But I was swallowing. I was swallowing a lot. I was swallowing air. I was using my neck muscles to swallow enough air to stay alive but not enough to talk. I wasn't going to suffocate—I was going to bleed to death. I had to forget about that. I couldn't do anything about it unless I could free my legs. If I could—

"Hey, there's somebody in here," someone yelled.

A man stuck his head in. "You okay? Are you hurt anywhere? Hey, buddy, are you okay?"

I looked at him and my mouth moved silently.

"Over here," he yelled over his shoulder. "I think he's in shock or something."

"Hold on. Hold on. Stay awake," they said.

Someone said it in the emergency room. I was hurting so bad I could hardly hear. I kept clenching my teeth against the pain and that made it difficult to swallow. I was so scared that just about all I could hear was my heart pounding. What I was hearing was fragments, pieces of conversations. Someone was taking my blood pressure. They had my wallet and something was said about calling my parents for permission to operate. They were doing something to my other arm—taking blood. A doctor was cutting away my shirt and asking questions I had no way of answering. Something was said about X-rays. I tried to ask if my neck was broken. Someone had said it was when they pulled me from the car.

"This is going to hurt a little," the doctor said, "but stick with me. It's going to feel a little strange for a minute but you'll be okay, just try to relax and let it happen."

He stuck something sharp into the base of my throat. I clenched my teeth and shut my eyes tight against the pain. I wanted to tell him it hurt, to stop, to stop cutting because it hurt and I couldn't stand the pain. I froze all over stiff and rigid like something dead. The cutting kept on in short little jerks, an instrument grabbing something and getting a piece of flesh with each grab.

"Almost over," he said.

I wanted to tell him that it was over, that I wasn't going to allow him to hurt me anymore, but he turned away to pick up something. Then he began pushing against my throat, pushing something into my throat. I gagged. Then again, and again. Oh, Jesus! My body began to jerk violently. To heave and jump.

I couldn't control it. I couldn't stop it and I couldn't swallow anymore. I couldn't breathe. I wanted to scream. I was so scared I started to faint, but I would die if I did. They'd told me I would. They told me to stay awake. Stay awake! Stay awake! Oh, Jesus. I couldn't breathe and I was going to faint.

Then it stopped. My body ceased its violent struggle.

"It's over. You'll be okay now," the doctor said. "You'll be able to breathe a little easier now."

I wanted to tell him this wasn't necessary, but he walked away. Someone I couldn't see began cutting my hair. I wanted to tell him, but I couldn't see him.

"Careful, he has a couple of bad cuts up here," a voice said.

All this wasn't necessary. If my neck was broken, all they had to do was give my head a yank. I'd seen it a thousand times in movies. They would grab a broken arm or leg and give it a yank, the guy would scream and pass out, and then he'd wake up okay. I might have to wear a cast, but if someone would just give my head one good yank it would stop the pain and I would be able to move again. I wanted to tell them that.

They finished cutting my hair and then they shaved my head.

"A little pin prick," someone said, and I felt the needle and in a moment my scalp began to tingle and then it went numb. I heard a drill but I didn't feel anything.

They took me to X-ray, and when they brought me back the doctor knelt down beside me.

"I've been in touch with your parents," he said. "They're on their way up here, but we're not going to be able to wait. You've injured your neck and we're going to have to operate to relieve the pressure. We're not going to be able to put you to sleep. I'm afraid you're too weak for that. We're going to use a local anesthetic. Now you're going to have to help us. We won't know exactly when we're touching the cord so you'll have to tell us."

I wanted to tell him that I didn't know what the cord was

and even if I did I wouldn't be able to tell him because I couldn't talk, but before I could let him know they were moving me again.

"Hold on. Hold on. Stay awake," they said.

Someone said it in the operating room.

"Now you let me know if it hurts," a woman sitting below me said, and I wondered how I was supposed to do that.

At first I tried to listen to everything that was being said, but I couldn't understand much of it, and what I did understand convinced me that I didn't want to know what they were doing. The local anesthetic had stopped the pain and I was suddenly very tired. I started drifting. I let the drugs carry me. I forgot about the people and what they were doing and where I was. I began to feel safe in a twilight world, a world void of pain and feeling.

My body erupted suddenly, without warning. It exploded into fire and the pain was more violent than anything I could ever have imagined.

I screamed. I screamed at the woman to stop them. Long, silent, agonizing screams.

"Are they hurting you?" she asked.

I blinked my eyes furiously.

"I think he's in pain," she told them, and the pain eased. The burning slowly ebbed. I heard the word "cord" spoken by someone.

It happened again. And again. There were bone chips. Sorry, but they had to be removed. It took forever. It took six hours. Each time I grew weaker and more tired. Each time I came closer to fainting and dying. Each time I cared less for life.

"Hold on. Hold on. Stay awake," I said to myself.

I said it in the recovery room where dreams beckoned. There were serpentine tubes everywhere—tubes running into both arms and my right foot. A tube dropped from the wall into an opening at the base of my throat. Another tube ran from beneath the sheet into a plastic bottle beside the bed. And

9

two small steel pins extending from my head held a chrome arch that had a nylon rope with metal weights attached to it.

I could stay awake as long as I kept the small comma-shaped crack in the ceiling in focus, but the crack kept changing into little animals and running off, leaving nothing but a stark white plane and dreams beckoning as compellingly as the sirens of legend.

If it ran again I wouldn't be able to find it. I was too tired. Too tired to search the ceiling anymore. If it ran off again I would die.

I didn't hear her say my name and I didn't see her until she leaned over me and broke my line of vision.

"Tom, your father and I are here," she said. She tried to smile but her lower lip began to tremble.

I started to smile, to let her know that everything was okay, not to worry. I wasn't going to sleep but my vision blurred. I tried to clear it. I tried to find the little crack but I couldn't. I tried to find the ceiling but I couldn't. I slipped into the gray-edged darkness of sleep.

When the anesthetic wore off, the pain began. It jerked me awake. It was more reflex than anything else that made me grip at the bed, but my hands did not move. The pain was growing rapidly, and a cold sweat began to run down my face, biting at my eyes. I clenched my teeth and tried to blink away the sting in my eyes. I tried to roll, to move away from the rising pain, but my body was not mine; it did not move. My heart began to pound as my sense of helplessness grew and each beat slammed into my neck like a hot steel hammer. I clenched my teeth harder and harder until the taste of blood brought with it a rising nausea, and still the pain came like some wild, living thing. I tried to cry out, to call for help, but the words gurgled out the tube in my throat, an inaudible rustle of air.

A furious panic seized me. I wanted to run screaming from the pain that tormented me but I couldn't run, I couldn't fight,

10

I couldn't even cry out in fear; and it was this—my utter and complete helplessness—that fired in me a deep, boiling fury. An anger, black and total, rose in me, and as it did the panic ebbed, for I was no longer helpless—I had found my weapon, but before I could use it I slipped back into darkness.

Floating back to consciousness, I didn't know if I had been out for minutes or hours or days. I knew I was hot. God! I was hot and sick. I knew I hurt. My neck hurt. It felt swollen, like a balloon ready to burst. The throbbing of my heart filled the balloon with each beat, filled it and stretched it. At any second it would burst. I knew it. I could see it. The balloon would burst! The air would rush out of it and I would die. I was rising and falling, spinning through the darkness into light, flashing, bursting light, and then into darkness again. The lights were spinning wildly, then exploding like fireworks at the fair, and far off in the distance I could almost make out the sound of the barker, "For one dime. One thin dime . . . "

It was the fall of the year, and nature had dressed herself in the yellow, red, gold of the season. The air had a kind of crisp, clean tingle that felt cool against the face, making a boy aware of the warmth within him and sometimes the loneliness. Rick had figured out that it wasn't the air or the colors or anything like that which made a person feel lonely in the fall. It was, he decided, sweaters. Fall was the time of the year when girls put on tight sweaters that showed their breasts to such advantage that a guy just naturally felt lonely. Richard Tucker and I had met in grammar school and had spent a lot of our time puzzling over the mysteries of life. The mysteries of breasts, of buttocks, of legs, of why girls said "no" most of the time and "yes" at the damnedest times.

Rick and I had come to the county fair hoping to get into the strip shows for the first time. Standing there before the judge, Rick carefully studied his own feet as I explained that we had climbed the fence only to keep from standing in line for such a long time, that we would be glad to pay. The judge

11

ran the fair and made a lot of money doing it, so he took it seriously. He knew Rick and me, as he knew most of the boys in our small town. "Since you don't want to call your fathers, I'll let you guard the fence," the judge said. "Get one of those heavy canes and keep anybody from coming over the west section. I'm not kidding with you boys. If anybody climbs over the fence, I'll lock you both up for trespassing. Do you understand me?"

"Yes, sir," I said. I thought the judge was taking the whole thing too seriously. "Can't we just pay you for a ticket and go on?"

"Son, you broke the law climbing in here. You break the law, you got to pay the penalty. Now, get out there," the judge said sternly. "And stay away from the girlie shows."

We spent the next several hours walking up and down the narrow, dark path between the back of the tents and the fence, stepping over the thick cables that snaked through the grass. Occasionally chasing a kid off the fence, we listened to the sounds of the rides blending like a giant calliope, the squeals and giggles of the girls. We smelled the wonderful, mysterious, once-a-year fragrance of the fairgrounds, felt the excitement and electricity and hated ourselves.

I saw him first. He wasn't a kid. He was big and mean-looking, straddling the top of the fence. I thought about letting him go. I didn't want to confront anyone who looked like that. The man's T-shirt was a second skin. His massive arms, covered with tattoos, threatened to burst the sleeves with each move. Then I thought of the jail and my father having to come get me out. "Hold it, buddy!" I said. "You can get a ticket down at the gate."

"I'd rather come in here," he said, swinging his leg in an arc to clear the fence.

I moved quickly, placed the tip of the cane on the man's chest and shoved hard. He fell backwards, landing with a thud. He was on his feet immediately, fists clenched, teeth bared.

12

"You little son of a bitch," he snarled, as he started over the fence again. When his hand was on the top strand of wire, I came down hard on it with the cane. With a yell of pain, he fell back again, "Goddamn you!" he growled, rubbing his hand.

"Look, mister, I don't care if you climb over or not," I said nervously. "The only reason I'm here is because they caught me climbing in. They're going to lock me up if I let anybody come in here. Go on over to the other side and climb in. There's a good place down there in the back, and there ain't nobody watching it."

"No. I'm coming in here," he said menacingly. "And I'm gonna whip your ass."

I looked nervously for Rick as the man started up the fence again. Just as his head cleared the top I hit him lightly across the nose, knocking him down again. He got up slowly, brushing himself off. He pointed his finger at me and said softly, "You stay right there, don't go anywhere, 'cause I'm gonna buy me a ticket and I'm gonna come cut your guts out."

As he walked off toward the gate, Rick came walking up. "Do you think he means it?"

"I don't know."

"Did you see the arms on that son-of-a-bitch? Did you see those tattoos?"

"Yeah, I saw 'em."

"Well . . . what are we gonna do?"

I shrugged. "What can we do?"

"I think we ought to forget about this fence business and go to the girlie show," Rick suggested.

"And what happens if we bump into him in there? Or, worse, what if he sees us and we don't see him?"

"Aw, he's crazy. He ain't gonna do nothing," Rick said. We turned our attention to a couple of kids trying to sneak in. We chased them off and continued to walk up and down the fence, keeping a wary eye on the gate.

"Here he comes!" Rick cried excitedly. "Goddamn, he looks like an ape! What are we gonna do?"

"I don't know," I said, trying to think. "Just wait and see what he does, I guess. But listen, stand kinda behind him and if I hit him, let him have it. I mean really unload on him."

"With a stick? You mean with this stick?"

"Hell, yes, I mean with a stick. If he's got a knife, I'm not about to get close enough to hit him with my fist."

"I've never hit anybody with a stick before."

"You think I have?" I said angrily.

The man's long fast strides carried him to within a few feet of me. He looked bigger and meaner now that there wasn't a fence between us. Rick moved beside him, slightly behind him. The man glanced at Rick, and Rick at me. He smiled a slow, evil smile and held out his left hand.

"I got my ticket," he said. "Now, you're gonna get yours." As he pulled his right hand from his pocket, the lights of the fair danced off a glittering steel blade. It had just cleared his pocket when I swung. I arced the cane high in the air and brought it down as hard as I could. Rick was a fraction of a second behind me.

A few minutes later, standing in the back row of the girlie show, Rick whispered, "Do you think we killed him?"

"I don't know," I whispered. "I didn't look back."

"I did. He was just lying there. I never hit anybody with a stick before. How hard did you hit him?"

"As hard as I could."

"Me too. Do you think he's dead?"

"No, I don't think so. I mean . . . I don't know. Anyway, we were just doing what the judge said. I was so damn scared, I had to hit him. My legs were shaking so bad I thought I was going to fall down any minute."

Rick seemed surprised. "You were scared too?"

"Yeah," I said nervously. "Let's get out of here."

As we walked out of the tent, I heard the barker far across

the midway. . . . "For one dime. One thin dime. One tenth of a dollar . . ."

A rocket exploded in the night sky and in my neck. The fireworks were beginning. I melted into the black sky, floating, drifting, spinning, the world alive with waterfalls of color . . . and pain . . . the deafening report of the rockets becoming the sound of my heart as it pounded in my ears, the heat of the explosions burning me, choking me until I fainted into a restless sleep filled with dreams.

2

IT WAS Christmas and my brother, Wayne, was there. The house was full of Christmasy things, with smells of evergreen and packages under the tree and a fire roaring in the fireplace. My mother was humming in the kitchen and acting secretive. She always acted that way at Christmas. Always coming in with packages, not saying anything, just smiling at us and going to the back of the house. I could see Wayne throwing his football, throwing it all wrong and having a grand time howling and yelling. But it wasn't Wayne anymore, it wasn't home anymore. It was the crowd at the ball game, and I was carrying the ball and running, running, running on an endless field until my legs quit and I fell and the crowd sighed.

There was Rick telling me he had it figured out. Rick was always figuring things out, mostly about girls and mostly wrong. He had figured out that the field was painted on a huge conveyor belt. The faster you ran, the faster it turned. You could never get to the end. You had to stop running and start jumping. You jump up and let the field, which was really a belt, pass under you. So, we were jumping up and down, up and down, out in the middle of a football field with the crowd confused and yelling at us. I hoped Rick was right because I didn't want to jump up and down and confuse everybody unless it was right. I was jumping up and down and yelling because my father had me by the arm spanking me with a belt that had football fields on it. "It wasn't right," he was saying. "It wasn't right to hit a little girl." But it was right. She had kicked me so I punched her in the eye, and I would do it again, even if my father did hit me with a football field. I would punch her again because I wanted to.

I wanted to because she wasn't little anymore. She was all grown up, and warm and soft, and I wanted her so bad. I wanted her so damned bad. I hated her and loved her and wanted her. I hated her for taunting me and hated myself for wanting her so much. I could never sleep at night, lying there thinking of what to say to her, how her breasts must look, what they must feel like. What anybody's must feel like. God! If I didn't find out soon, I would die, explode and die. Damn her! Damn her! I would like for her to suffer as I did all the nights I lay awake trying to see her in my mind, thinking of what she would look like, standing there with the moonlight filtering through her gown. I could see her, only it wasn't my room anymore, and her gown wasn't white with moonlight behind it. Why would she wear such a thing, all rough and black, with a hood? That's just what she would do. She would agree to come to my room, knowing what I had planned a thousand times, and she would wear a Halloween costume and laugh at me for my silly plans. But it wasn't her at all. I had seen him somewhere. I knew that hollow-eyed skull, that frozen smile, but I didn't know how I knew.

Dear God! Sweet Jesus! It was Death, and he had come for me. It wasn't time! It couldn't be time! I was eighteen, and nobody dies at eighteen. I hadn't lived yet, I was hardly born yet. I had not done one single thing that I wanted to do, and there was Death, telling me it was time. It was *not* time! Death was wrong. He would have to wait. Everybody would come to him. He wouldn't have to lift a finger. They would come. But he would not wait. He reached out a skeletal hand and grabbed me by the neck. The long bony fingers sank deep into the flesh, sending pain screaming through my body, violently yanking me awake.

My eyes opened to a spinning white blur that hurt my head and made me dizzy. I closed them again on a world full of sounds—hums, buzzes, squeaks, gurgles. It was probably the generator that ran the ferris wheel . . . but it couldn't be that . . . I wasn't at the fair. That was a long time ago, back home, and I wasn't at home. I didn't know where I was or what was happening to me. I couldn't open my eyes; it was hot and I was sick and hurt and confused. I didn't know if I was awake or asleep, alive or dead. Maybe I was dead! It was hot enough, and I hurt enough. Maybe I was dead and this was hell, and this was what it was going to be like for the rest of eternity. I had seen Death come for me, saw him reach out a bony arm with tattoos on it. But that couldn't be. Bones don't have tattoos, only flesh has tattoos, and Death had no flesh. I couldn't be dead. It wouldn't be like this. You wouldn't just start to burn. Somebody would point a finger at you first. Somebody would point a finger at you and yell, "Now you're going to get it, you good-for-nothing sinner! Now you're going to burn!" That's the way they would do it. Nobody would just start burning, so I must be alive. I didn't seem to have a body. How could I be alive, and not have a body? Why couldn't I talk or cry out if I was alive—unless I was asleep? I had seen my mother, I could remember that, so I must be awake. I saw her at Christmas, and she said she would be in the kitchen . . . no . . . that's not it. That's not what she said at all, and it's not Christmas. Where did I see her? It was a strange room, I could remember that. A room full of snakes. Was it snakes? No . . . no . . . it was tubes. That's right, it *was* tubes, and she said something about going outside. What was that noise? Was it a car? No . . . not exactly a car. Outside? Why would she go outside? Maybe Wayne was still outside throwing his football, she would have to go outside to get him. It could be a motorcycle, that noise. Of course, it's a motorcycle. It's Rick! That's it. It's beginning to make sense. It's Rick and his motorcycle. I was lying in the street and couldn't open my eyes, and Rick was roaring off, leaving me. . . .

It was dark, almost eleven o'clock, as Rick and I silently pushed the motorcycle up the side street. Rick had a summer job as a delivery boy for the drugstore, and they let him keep the motorcycle. We were full of nervous excitement, trying to be as quiet as possible. We had done it before and that's why we were nervous. If we were caught, if the workers were expecting us . . . but they wouldn't be. It had been weeks since we last did it.

The third-shift textile workers sat in long rows along the curb, waiting for the shrill whistle to call them to work. They sat with their feet in the gutter, the brown paper bags containing their lunch or breakfast held carelessly in their laps. Rick called them lintheads because of the cotton lint that clung to their hair after eight hours at the looms.

Easing the motorcycle around the corner, we climbed on. Rick fired the engine to life and opened the throttle. The scream of the engine shattered the night air. The motorcycle leaped forward, thundering down the gutter and the long row of workers who, in an attempt to get their feet out of the way, were falling backward, the women screaming and throwing their lunch bags in the air, the men, once recovered, cursing and shaking their fists. Rick was leaning into the wind as though he was in a race with life itself. I sat on the back, flapping my arms and legs and yelling at the top of my voice.

Neither of us saw the huge old woman standing at the far end of the row. She was waiting like an angry sow, one foot planted stubbornly in the gutter, the other on the curb. From her lunch bag she had taken a large, ripe tomato.

19

Rick saw her at the last moment and swerved slightly to miss her, just as she brought her chubby arm forward and threw the tomato with all her strength. She aimed for Rick, hoping to knock him off the motorcycle, but her aim was bad. The tomato sang by his head, almost nicked his ear, and landed squarely in my face. My legs flew up in the air and I rolled backward off the motorcycle, landing flat on my back in the street. I didn't know what had happened. I had not seen the stubborn old woman. I lay there in the street, stunned, not able to open my eyes because of the stinging acid of the tomato. My head hurt, and I was confused as I listened to the sound of the motorcycle speeding off into the night. . . .

Lying in the hospital, I waited for the lintheads to jump on me, to kick me and beat me and curse me. It all made sense, someone had hit me with something. Probably a brick. It felt like a brick. I was hurt, hurt bad, and Rick was leaving me. That couldn't be right. Rick wouldn't leave me. We had stood by each other all our lives. Rick would never leave me to face the lintheads alone. That was a long time ago. I could remember doing things since then. That happened before I went to college and I *did* go to college, so I couldn't still be lying in the road. Then what was that noise? Why couldn't I move or talk? Everything kept melting together, blurring out of focus and back into focus . . . changing . . . moving . . .

I was more confused than ever. I had to think, but I was too tired to think. I could feel it slipping away from me, the last bit of energy oozing out of me, and with it—life. I was floating, almost asleep. No. I must not sleep. Someone had told me not to sleep. If I slept, I would die. I had to stay awake. Maybe I was dreaming? Maybe I had fallen asleep and was dreaming and dying. I had to think. I couldn't think anymore. I didn't know anymore. I didn't care anymore. I let go. I stopped thinking and began drifting, floating across a thousand skies until a peaceful, restful sleep pulled me gently down into billowy clouds.

The pain had ebbed, settling into a constant, dull ache when I next awakened. Opening my eyes, I quickly shut them against the glare reflecting from the ceiling. Squinting, I opened them again, watching as the square white ceiling began rocking from side to side, made a complete turn, and continued slowly spinning. It made me dizzy, then sick. I closed one eye. The ceiling stopped spinning, rocked from side to side a few times, settled into its normal position. I was thirsty. I ran the tip of my tongue over parched, cracked lips, wondering where I was. My head was pulled back and held in a position that limited my vision to the ceiling and portions of the upper walls. I wondered if I was alone. I reopened my eye. The ceiling rocked. I closed it.

"Well, did you finally decide to wake up?" Mom asked, smiling down at me. I saw her for a second before my eye lost focus, found her again, lost her. I opened the other eye, blurring the image even more. When I closed it, the haze melted. I could see her. I started to speak, frowned, forgot what I was going to say. "You certainly slept long enough," she said.

Then I remembered what I wanted to say, but my lips moved in silence.

She placed her finger over the mouth of the tube in my throat.

"Try it now," she said gently.

"What time is it?" I asked. The sound came out a haggard whisper.

"Ten o'clock," she said, lifting her finger slightly.

"Friday?" I rasped; the word was thick and muffled.

"Sunday. You've slept almost three days."

My lips moved. She lowered her finger. "Was . . . was . . . there a . . . a motorcycle in here?"

She chuckled. "No. No motorcycle. You're in the hospital,

in Asheville." She lowered her finger, thinking I wanted to ask something else. I didn't. She continued, "A lot of your friends from college came by, Rick was here, and some people from the church. . . ."

I knew she was saying something but I couldn't make out what it was. Her voice was an echo at the far end of a tunnel. I began drifting again.

Awakening later, I was startled to see my father standing over me. Damn! I must have really messed up. My father never took time off from work. He worked six days a week—every week. He'd never taken a vacation and I couldn't remember him ever being out sick. But I realized that he must have been at the hospital for three or four days by now.

"Boy, you get enough sleep?" he said jokingly. He used the word "boy" affectionately, as he often did. It was his only expression of feeling for my brother and me.

"What you doing here?" I asked nervously.

"Your mother and I thought we ought to be here."

"Dad, I was just trying to get home. It was just an accident."

"I know," he said softly. "I know."

"I'll be okay. I can handle this. You didn't need to come all the way up here."

"Listen—" He leaned down as if to take me into his confidence and whispered, "I've been trying to get your mother off to myself for ten years. This little trip is going to do us a world of good." He straightened up and winked at me.

I was fully awake now. My vision was clear but my neck felt tight, bloated. I could feel each heartbeat above the ache. Mom came into vision as I cautiously asked, "What's wrong with me?" I saw the look she gave my father before he said, "You've fractured some bones in your neck."

"Why can't I move?"

"Well, the way I understand it," he explained, "when the vertebrae broke, they pressed against the spinal cord and that prevents the brain from getting its messages to the muscles."

There must still be some pressure, I thought. Things swell after surgery but as soon as that goes down . . . "How long will I be here?" I asked, barely making myself heard.

"Why? You got some plans?" he asked, trying to lighten the situation.

"I've got an interview next week."

"Well, let's not worry about that right now," Mom put in. My lips moved. Dad had lost the rhythm, lifting his finger instead of pressing it. "How long?" I asked. Mom looked at him and neither of them spoke for a moment.

"They're not sure, at least a couple of weeks," he answered.

Damn. If I was going back to college I had to earn the money during the summer. That interview was important. I had to get home. I was suddenly very tired. There was something I wanted to ask, but I couldn't remember what it was. I started slipping off again.

The pain woke me, building steadily in my neck. A cutting, stinging pain across my forehead and chin. I opened my eyes slowly, prepared for the glare that had greeted me before. At first I was confused, then frightened, by the gray and black speckled surface a few feet from my face. I had the feeling of being pulled toward it and yet I wasn't moving. I began to feel with my face. I raised and lowered my eyebrows, furrowed my brow, I moved my jaw from side to side and then I understood. Straps. They had strapped my head down. Why would they do such a thing? There was no reason I could think of. The pain in my neck was severe. I started to call out, then remembered the tube.

I studied the speckled surface but could not make it out. I searched frantically for the sight of someone who could help me or something recognizable that would explain it all. Nothing. Confusion and pain gave way to a wild, rampant panic that could find no expression. My heart pounded in my ears. I could not get my breath. My inability to release my panic brought on new waves of it until every fiber of my being screamed in agonized terror. I had to stop this! I had to get control of myself. I had to stop the fear that made me want to run screaming like a frightened child. I had to think. Think! Think! Think, you bastard, I screamed at myself. That's all you can do, so do it. All I had left was my mind and with this realization came an eerie calm. The same dispassionate lull had awaited me earlier in my flight from the relentless pain of the emergency room and surgery. A stoic, pacific acceptance that left only the cold, logical machinery of thought.

I studied the black and gray specks again—this time slowly, systematically eliminating one possibility after another. I felt relieved, giddy at first, then foolish that I had allowed myself to be frightened. It was the floor. I was on my stomach. The straps were supporting me. The understanding did not lessen the pain. It would not ease until they turned me over. I wondered if it would be minutes or hours before they came. Maybe it would be days. Maybe they were going to leave me like this every other day. One day on my stomach, one day on my back. Dear God. I couldn't stand the pain that long. Not for days at a time, they couldn't do that. Surely they wouldn't. If I thought about it the pain would get worse. I had to think of something else. I could not concentrate. I tried. I tried remembering lyrics to popular songs but was unable to escape into the thought. I tried multiplying numbers but lost track when the numbers grew too large. Poetry. I liked poetry but could not remember the words to any poems. I had memorized many, for class and for myself, but I could not recall them now. The pain kept crowding me, pushing me, it kept coming, coming, coming. Enough was enough, by God. I was infuriated by the thought that I had done all I could and it still came. Pain suddenly took form and shape, and became a personal antagonist that I had tried to avoid, had tried to escape and, at last, had tried to ignore. But it would not be ignored, it kept coming at me, so now I would deal with it. No more

24

games, no more running. It was a simple contest. I had tried to be conciliatory but was not allowed to be, so now I would fight. I would use my hate, my frustration, my rage. I would unleash all the wrath in me and I would annihilate it. I would do it by force of will. I would not be pursued like this, pushed and tormented like this.

I would deal with the pain across my forehead first. Along the edge of the strap cutting into me the pain was well defined. I imagined it as a fiery red line. I would erase it just as I would a line drawn by a pencil. I got a clear picture of it in my mind. I imagined it to be six inches long and held the image in my mind, hating it. Then I cut an inch off the end and held the thought. I savored the relief over one inch of my forehead, relished the coolness of it, putting any thought of the pain in my neck and across my chin out of my mind, holding onto the image of a fiery red line five inches long. I cut off another inch. Relief. A four-inch line.

I had pushed it to two inches when they came. I didn't hear them, and was first aware of them when I felt something press the back of my head. They were going to turn me. No! Not yet! I was winning! They could wait a minute! I needed this victory. They could wait. Suddenly without warning, without a word, I was spun rapidly. My neck exploded. The spinning motion stopped abruptly, leaving me sick to my stomach. I felt a hot, searing pain deep in my neck—a hot gushing, a terrible burning, an awful fire that spread into my shoulders. I closed my eyes and clenched my teeth in agony. As the straps were lifted from my face the relief was exquisite. The air on my chin and forehead was deliciously cool. The pain in my neck began to subside. I opened my eyes and saw her standing there.

"Are you all right?" she asked.

My lips moved in silent response.

"Are you in pain?" the woman asked, watching more intently.

25

Again I answered her silently.

"You'll have to speak up," she snapped. "I can't hear you."

Frustration flared into rage as I sought some means of expression. Mom was at my side immediately, explaining that in order for me to speak it was necessary to place a finger on my throat.

"Uh," the woman grunted. "Does he want something for pain?"

Mom placed a finger over the tube.

"Why, you stupid bi— . . ."

Mom quickly raised her finger. "Maybe you'd better leave," she told the woman.

I glared at the woman as she left the room, then I glared at my mother as she began to carefully bathe my raw forehead. I was furious with the woman, with my mother, and with my helplessness, and I needed to vent that anger. I tried frantically to catch her eye but she avoided my heated gaze. When she had finished bathing my face she began gently to rub a soothing lotion over the irritated skin. She looked down at me shyly, smiled, and shook her head slowly. "Uh-uh," she murmured, "not until you calm down."

I scowled at her and thought about faking it, but just then she reached out and touched the small crescent-shaped scar on the bridge of my nose and smiled knowingly. There wasn't any way I could fake being calm, not with that scar. It would be glowing red as it always did when I was angry.

"You shouldn't get so upset," she said, turning her attention once again to the lotion. "She didn't know. She's only an aide and she just didn't know." Spending more time than necessary rubbing on the lotion, she kept at it until the red hue of anger drained from my face and the vein in my forehead no longer threatened to rupture itself. "Now," she said, placing her finger over the tube.

"What kind of bed am I on?" I asked. I knew if I mentioned the aide Mom would take her finger off the tube.

"It's not a bed at all," she explained. "It's called a Stryker frame. It's a metal frame with canvas over it. There's another one just like it over here in the corner. They just lay it on you and hook it at both ends. Kind of makes a big sandwich out of you and then it's flipped over and the part you were lying on is removed. Your father can explain it better. He'll be back in a few minutes."

"How often will I have to turn?"

"They want you on your stomach one hour out of four. So you stay on your back for three and on your stomach for one."

I frowned at the thought.

"You have to be turned or you'll get pressure sores," she added.

"Pressure sores?"

"Yes. Sores caused by lying in one position for a long time."

The thought wasn't a pleasant one and that brought to mind something else. "I meant to ask you. What happened to the guy who picked me up, the driver?"

"He went home. They didn't even have to admit him."

"He didn't get hurt at all?"

"Well, he was scratched up some. He was thrown out, thrown clear."

My father came back into the room just then and we talked for a while. He told me who had been to see me, read the telegrams. He told me I had made the front page of my home-town paper.

"Don't let it go to your head," Mom warned. "It was right beside an article on the new sewer system."

There was a movement behind them. "Would you excuse us, please," Dr. McKinnon said, entering the room, his nurse close behind him.

He handed the chart to his nurse and was already examining the sutures in my head as my parents made their way out of the room.

"Do you remember me?" he asked, looking at me unsmiling and placing a finger on my throat.

27

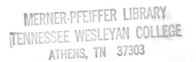

It was hard to believe the man standing by my bed, dressed in a blue pin-striped suit, was the same man I had last seen in the recovery room. He was a small man who looked to be somewhere in his late forties, but he'd been dressed in the baggy green uniform common to the operating room. His short, light-brown hair had been matted from hours beneath an operating room cap and had framed a round expressionless face. His eyes had been sharp and intelligent but showed the strain of six hours in surgery, and exhaustion had hung about him like an ominous fog. His face was still expressionless.

"Yes, I remember you," I told him.

"The last few days have been rough, I know, but I think the worst is over. Things should begin to ease up a bit now," he said as he continued his examination. He studied the tube at the base of my throat, probed, poked, grunted, and instructed his nurse to make a notation on his chart. He was at the foot of the bed for a while, out of my range of vision. "I'm going to prick you lightly with a pin and I want you to tell me when you feel it," he instructed. The nurse put her hand on my throat.

"Now?" he asked.

"No."

"Now?"

"No."

"And now? How about here?" he asked, working his way up to my chest, across my shoulder, and down my arms.

"Nothing, I don't feel anything," I told him.

The doctor thought for a moment as he folded the pin and put it away. "This will hurt a little, just hold on," he said, as he slid his hand beneath my neck. Then he pressed his hand flat against it and lifted up. The light went out suddenly. Then it came back again, spinning dizzily in the ceiling. I swallowed hard, forcing down the bitter bile that rose in my throat. I blinked away the ragged edges of unconsciousness that clouded my vision. Liquid fire ran out of my neck into my shoulders. My arms twitched involuntarily.

"Okay, just hang on. It'll be over in just a minute," he reassured me, as he retracted his hand. He nodded to his nurse and she quickly injected a pain-killing drug. "That should help ease it. We'll check with you later," he said as they left the room.

The drug began taking effect and the pain was subsiding when my parents returned. We talked until my words became thick and muffled and I drifted off to sleep.

3

EACH day I waited for movement to come, for feeling to return, and the passing days began to take on a sameness as I grew accustomed to their routine and ritual. The early mornings were usually busy with breakfast, a bath, the changing of bed linens, and Dr. McKinnon's daily examination. I was left relatively undisturbed the remainder of the day and night except for blood pressure and temperature readings. The time I spent on my stomach was always agonizing, with pain waiting like a cunning predator.

When there was no pain, it was like being an inch tall and trapped in a fallen suit of armor. I could move around inside of it, down the hollow tubular legs, across the cavernous stomach, and up to the head, where I could peer out the eye holes and make myself heard out of the slit of a mouth, but I could not escape nor could I move the fallen giant. I began to realize how alone each of us is. I began to understand that there is a part of us that is forever alone—a part that cannot be reached by another human being, regardless of the amount of love between them, regardless of the amount of compassion or concern. I had to meet pain alone, and one day I would meet death the same way. I would have to take that journey from life to whatever waits on the other side completely alone. All those gathered about me, all those who loved me, would not be able to climb into this body to quell the terror or experience the peace. There seemed to me something basic about that knowledge—a truth, beautiful and sad.

I began to realize other things. The swelling had gone down, there was no longer any pressure on the spinal cord, and still I could not move, so it wasn't a simple matter of removing the pressure. Nothing else was going to change. They had done all they were going to do with surgery, the swelling and the pressure were gone, my neck was the way it would always be, there were no changes to wait for any longer. And yet McKinnon waited for something, he looked for something each day, so there must be time, however long or short, there must be a period of time before return begins. I didn't ask because he might be looking for something else. I didn't ask because time might have run out and I didn't want to know. I didn't ask because I didn't want to hear the word "permanent." As long as I didn't hear it, I didn't have to face it. As long as I didn't hear it, there was hope with each waking.

I turned my efforts toward moving a toe. I began to concentrate on that single effort before time ran out. I began to concentrate so totally that I seldom responded to the sound of voices. It was necessary for the nurses to touch my face in order to get my attention, and even this method, on occasion, had to be repeated several times before I became aware of them.

It was during one of these periods of concentration that I felt a hand on my face and opened my eyes to see my father standing over me. It was my eighth day in the hospital.

"Your Aunt Myrtle is here," he said with a hint of resignation. "You feel like seeing her?"

"Yeah, I guess," I said, then the thought hit me. "Dad, have you told me everything—everything that's wrong with me?" I made no attempt to hide the alarm.

"Yes, we've told you everything. Why? Is something wrong?"

"I think I'm busted up inside."

"What's wrong?" he asked with mounting concern.

"I—I haven't taken a leak in eight days."

He looked surprised at first, and then he broke into a broad smile.

"You've got a catheter."

"You mean there's a—a tube—in my—?"

"Yes." He laughed.

"Will it—I mean, will I—you know—does it—?"

"Oh, no," he said, shaking his head. "It doesn't affect anything. It's a common procedure. So you'll be just as good"—he laughed—"or just as bad as ever."

I was relieved to hear that.

Just then Mom came in with her older sister from Ohio, Myrtle Joyner. Myrtle began to cry before she had taken more than a step or two into the room. I watched as she wiped at the tears and fought to regain her voice. I'm stoic by nature and tend to consider public displays of emotion demeaning and distasteful. But Aunt Myrtle, I knew, had come all the way from Ohio for just this moment, and I would not spoil it. I waited patiently for her to act out her drama.

"Oh, Tom, ohhh, my dear Tom," she moaned at last.

"Hello, Aunt Myrtle."

"My poor, dear Tom," she got out before her voice gave way to sobs.

I waited.

"I'm sorry. I'm so sorry."

"I know."

"It isn't fair! It just isn't fair! You were always such a good boy," she wept. "Why? Why did this have to happen to you? It isn't right."

This question had never occurred to me. I thought about it and found that it was a question I could not ask myself seriously. "There isn't any why, Aunt Myrtle. It was an accident. Accidents happen. There is no why."

32

She launched into a predictable emotional oration. I didn't want to listen. I thought about her standing there full of health and never asking why. It seemed to me that if people questioned life's tragedies, then they should also question the absence of them. She should demand that God explain the reason for her good health when people her age were dying every day from a thousand causes.

Myrtle had stopped talking and seemed to be waiting for a reply. I wondered what the question was. "Uh-uh," I grunted and tried to looked interested. I knew immediately that it was the wrong answer. She frowned at me, then turned a puzzled look toward my parents, who were ashen.

"No, dear. I asked if you felt like telling me what happened," she repeated.

"When?" I asked, having no idea where the conversation had led or what she was talking about.

"In the accident, dear. How did the accident happen?"

"Oh," I sighed, and understood my parents' expressions. This question had been carefully avoided.

I told her how the man who gave me a lift kept running off the shoulder of the road. It scared me and I decided to get out, but since the man had been kind enough to pick up a soaking wet stranger, I didn't want to hurt his feelings by telling him that he was a lousy driver. So I made up a story about visiting relatives in the next town, five miles ahead. A few minutes later, the man ran off the shoulder and lost control.

"So, you see, if I hadn't been raised to be so polite"—I cut my eyes accusingly toward my mother—"I wouldn't be in this mess."

Mom threw up her hands in mock distress. "I knew it!" she exclaimed. "I knew you would find some way to blame me for it. I'm just surprised it took you this long."

In that moment I loved her more than I ever had. I loved her for not being Aunt Myrtle, for not wringing her hands in despair, and for being able to joke even now. I loved her for

33

taking her finger off a tube and refusing to put it back on, for keeping the tremendous emotions of the time private. I loved her for being what she always had been and for refusing to let time or circumstances affect the easy rapport we had always enjoyed.

"You don't expect me to take the responsibility for this, do you?" I said.

"Knowing you, no! But why me? Why hang it on me?"

Myrtle had watched the exchange in horrified amazement. She had never understood the relationship between my mother and me. To her, the situation called for emotion, for reflection, for spiritual interpretation. "God loves you!" she exclaimed.

"I know," I said, somewhat startled by her outburst.

"You must not blame God for this, Tom."

"I don't," I replied, cutting my eyes toward Mom.

Mom rolled her eyes toward the ceiling.

"It's a miracle you're alive at all," Myrtle said.

I couldn't think of anything to say to this.

"There has to be a reason you're still here. God has a purpose for you. He's left you here for a reason."

"Oh, no, you don't. You're not going to stick me with that. That's a terrible burden to put on a person, and I don't plan to lug it around."

"Whatever are you talking about?"

"Divine destiny. If I start thinking that I'm alive because God has something for me to do, then all my life I'll be wondering what it is. No thank you."

As soon as I said it, I knew I had made a mistake. I should have agreed with everything she said. Now she wanted to discuss religion. She launched into her diatribe with the fervor of a recent convert and the cadence of a hell-fire-and-damnation revivalist. I let my mind wander, and her voice trailed off in space. I recalled a thought I had had earlier.

The idea was new to me. I had thought I understood the separation of mind and body, but the full extent of that separation had just become apparent to me. Tom Helms was perfectly all right. Nothing had changed in my life. I was exactly as I had always been. I felt the same. My thoughts were the same. My desires were the same. My hunger was the same. I still thought of girls as I always had and wanted them in the same way. I still saw beauty and ugliness and was moved by them. I felt the same fears, the same anger, the same compassion, the same needs, the same sorrow, the same joy. Absolutely nothing had changed for me except that someone had stolen my body. Somebody had picked me up and set me down outside my body. And it was this thought that intrigued me. Nothing was wrong with me. *I* wasn't paralyzed. The body lying in bed was—but I wasn't. I had always thought of that body as being me, but now I knew it wasn't. It had very little to do with me really, except for the fact that I was trapped in it. It was like being in a car that would not run anymore. In fact, it had no more to do with me than my car did. Thinking about it now, it seemed to me that a car was exactly what it was—a method of getting from one place to another. My car had stopped running, and I was locked inside. The truth of the thought fascinated me. I immediately applied it to everyone and saw life in a ridiculous panorama. Instead of a body, each person was born into a car and spent his life trapped in it. There were all kinds of cars—grand touring models, sleek sports models, average cars, and super cars. Some were shiny and new, some old and rusty, some ran swiftly and smoothly and were capable of intricate maneuvers, while others clunked and sputtered along, threatening to quit at any moment. Some unlucky souls got defective models at birth, but they were stuck with them and had to make life's journey the best way they could. You could never trade in your car. If you wrecked it, that was just too bad, you did not get a new one. There were body shops along the way, but they were limited in what they could do. They could repair some things and patch others, but there weren't very many parts that they could replace.

If you lost a wheel, for instance, you simply had to limp along. When a car was beyond repair, finished, the driver left it to be buried in a junkyard and went to some place where there were no cars. No one was sure where this was.

It was a strange world I saw, but the most curious thing, it seemed to me, was the value system that had grown up around the cars. Almost everything was geared to the cars and almost nothing to the drivers. Drivers were liked or disliked, their company sought or avoided, according to the size, shape, or color of their car. Drivers got very excited if a car had big bumpers or moved a certain way. There were actual cases of cars that met, fell in love, and got married without ever having looked inside to see who was driving, only to find later that they did not like the driver of the car at all. Even the color of the cars had great significance. It didn't matter who was driving, certain-colored cars were inferior and that was the way of it. The car was the thing. One simply did not have time to go around looking into cars to see who was driving. It was unpleasant and confusing. There did not seem to be any reason or logic behind it. Some small cars were driven by giants; and dull, uninteresting drivers, at times, had huge, grand cars. Some spectacularly beautiful cars could have stupid, ugly drivers while beautiful, complicated people went around in rusty wrecks.

I looked up in time to see Myrtle turning to leave. She was weeping again. I hoped I had done nothing to upset her. Then, remembering how much she enjoyed emotion, I wondered if I should hope I *had* done something to upset her.

On Saturday, the tenth day, Dr. McKinnon removed the sutures from my head and neck and was in the process of extracting the tube from my throat. It was a simple procedure which involved severing a single stitch on either side of the tube and sliding it from the trachea. I watched him carefully as I always did. I liked the unsmiling Dr. McKinnon, although I had never been able to engage him in conversation beyond

36

the answers I received to my constant questions concerning my condition. I was aware of Dr. McKinnon's reputation. His skill and ability were unquestioned, his dedication to his patients was legendary, but he was considered cold and unfeeling, ruthless at times, demanding always. To my way of thinking, this was ideal. Friendship was not necessary; confidence and trust were. I considered Dr. McKinnon an ally who shared a common struggle—an ally whose skill and knowledge would weigh heavily in the outcome of that struggle.

Dr. McKinnon dropped the tube on the medical tray and placed a Band-Aid over the incision.

"Doc, how come I can breathe if I'm completely paralyzed? I mean, why aren't my lungs paralyzed?"

Dr. McKinnon looked down sideways at me. His eyes seemed to probe, to measure. He took in a breath and exhaled deeply. "Well," he began, "breathing is controlled by the chest muscles, which are segmental from the thoracic levels. Your diaphragm, the muscle between your stomach and your chest, is supplied by the nerves that come off at C-three on four and—"

"That's the third and fourth vertebrae down from the skull, right?" I interrupted.

Dr. McKinnon nodded.

"And that's where my injury was?"

"Yes, C-three on four. Now, an injury at C-three pretty well knocks out the diaphragm, so you don't have any diaphragm function. It's a complete motor paralysis. The patient arrives not breathing—dead. This is the unusual thing in your case. We just don't know why function in this particular area was continued."

"Okay," I said. And then I decided to ask. "The other thing I don't understand is—if I was paralyzed because of pressure on the cord, and you removed that pressure, why can't I move?"

Dr. McKinnon looked at me expressionlessly. His eyes slipped over my face as if to memorize it. He looked down at the floor for a moment, then rested his tired, brooding eyes on me. "Well, with most patients, the force that causes the fracture, the breaking of the bone, the dislocation, applies a force to the spinal cord which causes disruption in the cord. The cord may look perfectly normal, it may be swollen, it may have hemorrhage in it, it may look grossly disrupted, or it may be literally torn into. In those situations, of course, we don't expect any recovery. Where the cord looks normal, but there is complete paralysis, both motor and sensory, so there's no feeling and no movement, no reflexes below the level of the injury—these people usually do not get any recovery at all. Now, if this is caused by pressure on the cord, we remove that pressure, like a disc that's slipped out and pressing the cord, or a piece of bone that's pressing on the cord. Sometimes, if we remove that pressure, things will get better. That's the situation in your case."

I chewed my lower lip as I heard the words echo and reecho down long empty corridors. *Sometimes, if we remove that pressure . . . sometimes . . . sometimes.* The impact of the words stunned me. I felt an aching dismay, a heavy, pressing weight.

"Then you can't tell me that in so many weeks I'll have my arms back, and so long after that my legs? There's no guarantee that I'll get anything back."

Dr. McKinnon looked away and paused for a long minute before he spoke. When he did, his tone was softer, warmer. "No, I can't make any promises. There are no time schedules and no guarantees. But I can tell you that just because you haven't had any return in ten days doesn't mean you won't. There's still room for hope. It's still relatively early. We'll know a lot more about what to expect in the next few weeks. I want a physical therapist to start passive exercises on you in a week or so. You have excellent muscle tone and I would like to prevent as much atrophy as possible. So, let's just hang on and see what develops over the next two or three weeks."

I lay with my eyes closed for a while after Dr. McKinnon

38

left. I had hoped that the news would be good, but in a way it didn't matter what they thought. It didn't really make any difference.

When I opened my eyes I saw my mother standing beside me, holding on to my arm with both hands. Her eyes were brimming with tears as she pressed her lips into a thin, quivering, sad smile.

"Oh, hey, now. Come on, Mom." I winked at her. "I'll be okay. I kinda figured something like this. It's just going to take a little longer, but we'll get there. You'll see. So, come on now. Don't let 'em get to you."

"Oh, they're not getting to me." She wiped at her eyes with the back of her hand. "I was just worried about you. I guess I should have known better." She smiled. "Tom, do you know what I pray for every night? Every night I ask the Lord to give you strength. That's all. Strength. I know you'll do the rest if He'll just give you the strength. I want you to pray too. Will you? Will you say a prayer each night?" she pleaded.

"I do pray, Mom. But listen to me. I'm going to get out of this. I'm going to beat it. I know it. I don't think it or feel it. I *know* it! I know it more surely than I've ever known anything. I want to tell you something."

I told her how I found God one summer day long ago beneath a sky of deep azure blue, a blue that comes to the south only in late summer. Since that day that rare deep blue had come to hold a special significance for me, inspiring in me a feeling of oneness with God, a serenity, a promise. I told her how I was staring up from the stretcher as they pulled me from the ambulance. In that moment before the pelting rain forced me to close my eyes, I saw in the dark, storm-filled clouds a small patch of deep, azure blue and I knew I was all right.

"I guess some people would say that's grasping at straws."

"No, I don't think so," she said, smiling. "You and Rick have always kidded each other about omens. Maybe this is a real one."

"Why not." I chuckled. "If the ancients could see the future in chicken bones, I can find hope in a blue sky."

That night in the brooding darkness of my room and my soul, I wondered about the nagging, persistent, indefinable current of anger that coursed through me. Not the flaring rage that met frustration or the steadfast wrath that faced down pain, but something more and something less. This anger had no target, no direction, yet it lived beneath the rest, lurked and hid and waited for the darkness, the quiet solitude, and was always there. It came with exhaustion, made itself felt just before sleep, and waited patiently for the first moments of early-morning consciousness. I had wondered about it often, but now I came to understand it. It was death's attempt to cheat me that angered me. It was the fact that I had come so close to dying while I was still preparing for life that aroused in me such a bitter resentment.

I didn't like school, had never liked it, but I had gone on beyond high school to college because everyone told me it would open up new vistas, add to life an understanding, bring with it a broadening. And I had listened. Life would be better, they said, taste sweeter, mean more, if only I would postpone it long enough to acquire the mental tools necessary to harvest its bounty. And I had heeded their counsel. Heeded it not for myself, because life was already full and sweet for me the way it was. No, I had taken their charted course to happiness not for myself, but for those I would one day love. I didn't want to look into the pleading face of a child or a wife one day and have to admit that I lacked the skill or knowledge to tear from the world the things they desired—the things that were supposed to make life more than it was.

I loved life. Life was beautiful, mysterious, wonderfully intoxicating. Life was to be lived—not prepared for, lived. And I had lived it, felt it, loved it in every way I had known—denying myself one thing only: the one thing that life demands of those that understand it, the simple indisputable command that it be shared. This was what I wanted most and this was what I had postponed. This was what life was all about, to care totally, to need absolutely, and to share—above all, to share. I had never allowed myself to care deeply for any of the eager young girls because I was not prepared yet to give myself completely. And now death had tried to cheat me. But I would not be cheated out of loving the way I needed, caring the way I wanted, sharing the way I must. I would know these things, I must. Were I to die without knowing them, my life would have been void of meaning, a time spent without purpose. No, death would not cheat me. I would live!

4

SHORTLY after noon on the following day, my father left for home. Because I was still not able to summon a nurse when I needed help, Mom remained with me. She was sitting by my bed, reading. I was buried in concentration, locked in a struggle with my body, determined to supplant the function of nerves and coerce muscles to react by force of will. She did not watch me at these times. My efforts seemed to her to be almost supernatural, otherworldly, creating in her an eerie feeling that was uncomfortable and disconcerting. I would lie for hours as if in a peaceful sleep, my breathing shallow and regular. Then, suddenly, with no change in the rhythm of my breathing or my expression, beads of sweat would cover my face, building in such profusion as to discolor the sheet beneath my head as it collected the only fruits of my labor.

The door opened slightly and Rick Tucker stuck his head in and glanced around the room.

He was shorter than I, broad-shouldered and solidly built. It seemed he had always been the same size. His thick rust-brown hair hung loosely on his forehead, and his deep-set, brooding eyes appeared always on the verge of tears. This, along with his cleft chin and the slight scar on his left cheek, gave him the appearance of one who suffered life's tragedies with silent dignity—when, in fact, he suffered not at all. The eyes he had inherited from his mother, the chin his father, and the scar was my contribution. He had acquired it shortly after I had been knocked off the motorcycle. To prevent such a thing from happening again, Rick had purchased a plastic windshield for the bike. I was working that summer, helping my father on his laundry truck, and was sitting on the loading platform when he came riding down the street. He held out his left arm, the fist clenched, the middle finger extended, and grinned at me. I grinned back, the plastered-on grin of a clown, and it was this—my lack of reaction—that held his attention. My reactions were always immediate. I would return the gesture or a shouted obscenity, but I would not sit there grinning. Rick did not see, as I did, the taxi in front of him stop for the traffic signal. His arm was still extended, his attention focused on my grin, when he rammed into it. He landed on the trunk of the taxi, sat there brushing pieces of the plastic windshield off himself, and waited for the cab driver's wrath. He glanced at me still sitting on the platform, my left hand clenched, the middle finger extended, the frozen smile now one of genuine delight.

Looking up from her book, Mom said, "Richard, well, come in, come on in."

"Hi, Mom." Rick whispered. "Is he asleep?"

"No, he's awake. Tom, look who's here."

"Hey, man, how you doing?" Rick whispered.

When I saw his expression, I quickly changed my smile into a feigned grimace. Holding the pained look a moment, I relaxed the muscles of my face and said through clenched teeth, "That was a bad one, really bad." Behind him, Mom smiled and knew what was coming. She slipped out of the room silently.

"You all right?" Rick asked, with mounting concern.

"I . . . I'll be all right . . . in a minute," I said. I clenched my teeth again violently, closed my eyes tight, furrowed my brow as though I was struggling with unspeakable pain. I opened my eyes wide, staring at him. He looked frantically around the room for Mom. I opened my eyes even wider, trying hard to look confused. "I know you! I've seen you before."

"Of course you know me," he said, reassuringly.

"Don't try to pull that on me. I know who you *really* are." He frowned.

"You're—you're—" I tried to continue, but his expression of concerned confusion caused me to burst into laughter.

He flushed with embarrassment. "You ass. You goddamn ass. Can't you ever be serious?"

"I can't help it." I got out through my laughter. "If you could see your face."

"Well, what do you expect? This is serious, so I figured I'd look serious."

"It's not that serious. I'm not dead. I swear, if I was lying in a casket, that's exactly the look you would be wearing."

He rolled his eyes toward the ceiling with a look of disgust.

"Everybody comes in here with the same look and they all say, 'How are you, son.' They all call me son. Then I say 'fine,' because that's all they want to hear. They don't have time to listen to all that's wrong with me, and besides, if I told them I didn't feel fine, they wouldn't know what to say. Then they tell me that so-and-so said hello and that they're praying for me. When they ask if I need anything, I say 'no.' Then they tell me to keep up the good work and to keep my spirits up. Then they tell Mom that I'm a fine boy, *a fine boy,* and that they couldn't do what I'm doing. What the hell am I doing anyway? Lying here saying 'fine, fine,' all day—big deal. And then you come in and start the same crap."

"Well, I don't know how you're doing, but you don't look worth a damn." Taking a close look at my head, he added, "Man, you can't ever go bald. You look awful. Really bad."

"Oh, yeah?"

"Yeah. I'm going to sit down before I get depressed."

"I can't see you if you sit down."

"So? You know what I look like and that scar in the top of your head is going to make me sick," he said, stretching out in the overstuffed chair.

"Scar?" I cried with alarm. "What scar? They didn't tell me about any scar. They told me I had tongs in my head. Now you tell me I'm scarred. Oh, my God, I can't take any more."

Rick tensed for a moment, then said, "Don't start that. You shit! Don't start that again. I'll leave. I'll get up and walk out of here."

"Okay, okay. So I know about the scar. I know about the tongs. I know about the neck. I know about the tube in my pecker. I know—"

"The tube in your pecker?" he exclaimed. "You got a tube in your pecker?"

"No, I walk down to the bathroom."

"Damn! I bet that hurt."

"I can't feel anything. You could cut my leg off with a pair of nail clippers and I wouldn't even know it."

"Oh, yeah. I forgot," he said. "Damn—a tube."

"It's just the injustice of it all," I said, trying to sound as much like a girl as possible. "For eighteen years I've fought and scratched to hold on to my—my virginity, my honor, saving myself for marriage. And now, to have it end like this. Oh, the cruelty of it all. To be struck down in my youth, the flower of my girlhood. To be ravaged. To be violated by an insensitive rubber tube. Torn from my girlish fantasies and cast into womanhood before my time. Oh, the shame of it, the absolute shame. Dead. My dreams are dead. What man would have me? Ruined. Struck down. Stained. Life is just too, too cruel. I was a flower that never had a chance to blossom. And now there's only one thing left to do."

"Suicide!" he suggested eagerly.

"No! Not suicide. Something better—I mean, worse, much worse. I'll become one of those—those creatures of the night. A woman of easy virtue. A prostitute. Oh, woe is me. To fall to such a lowly state. Who would have thought it? Who would ever have thought I could come to this?"

"Me," Rick said, bursting into laughter. "Reckon you're a good lay?"

"Absolutely one of the best. Of course, I can't bring my best moves to it, being paralyzed and all." There was a sudden surge of pain. I closed my eyes and clenched my teeth. I tried not to let Rick see it, but my face twisted into a grimace as I tried to fight back the pain by force of will. When it passed and I opened my eyes, Rick was standing by the bed.

"Can I do anything? Get a nurse or something?"

"No. It comes and goes. I'm okay."

"What do the doctors say?"

"They say it'll ease up."

"No, I mean about moving. When will you be able to start moving things again?"

"They don't know. I've got a feeling they don't think I'll move again—ever. They say I should have died and I didn't, and now they don't know what the hell to expect."

"Fuck a bunch of doctors. They don't know what the hell they're doing anyway," he spat out. "What do *you* say?"

"I'll make it. I'll get out of this."

"Damn right you will, damn right," he said excitedly. "That's what I wanted to hear. You can do it. I know it. You didn't die, did you?"

"Nope."

"Well, you're not going to stay paralyzed forever either."

"No, they're not going to stick old Tom in a bed for the rest of his life. I told you I'll make it. I guaran-damn-tee it. So calm down. I don't need any pep talk."

He frowned, then shrugged. "I wasn't giving that pep talk for you." We were quiet for a while. Then he said wistfully,

"Man, I sure wish you were home. Concord is really dead."

"Did you get a job?"

"Yeah, I'm working out at the dairy. Jimmy's working out there too, or was."

"Jimmy Casteen?"

"Yeah. I've got to tell you this. You're going to love it," he said with a big grin. "We wear rubber knee boots and carry rubber hoses with a piece of lead in the tip—sort of tap the cows on the butt and they'll move. Well, old Casteen goes into this pen and starts spreading straw, and he's over in the corner and when he turns around there's this bull standing there looking him eyeball to eyeball."

"And he panics, right?"

"Now wait a minute," he said. "This ain't no ordinary run-of-the-mill bull. It's some real expensive prize bull that they're renting for breeding. I mean, they don't even own the damn thing. Well, old Jimmy goes kind of stiff and just stands there scared shitless. Then the bull lowers his head to take a bite of straw or something, and Jimmy thinks he's going to charge, so he whips out his hose and *whap*—he smacks the fucker right across the head. Well sir, that damn bull lets out a bellow, starts rocking from side to side, and then just falls over—dead, for all we know.

"The foreman comes running up yelling for somebody to call for the vet, and there's this big-ass bull just laying there and Jimmy standing there mumbling to himself—you know the way he does when he gets nervous." Rick laughed. "And it turns out that the bull was just knocked out. Old Jimmy had flat cold-cocked him. So they fired him, but he said he didn't give a damn because he was going to quit anyway."

We were quiet again, lost in reverie. I was remembering that summer day a year before. Rick and Jimmy and I were riding around in Rick's old Ford coupe, trying to fill up the day. On the floor there was a watermelon left from the adventures of the previous night, and the huge butcher knife we

47

had used to open our stolen treasure. We often went to the incinerator to shoot the large rats that made their homes among the piles of garbage. We knew the workmen sat at the opening of the building at the same time each day, eating their lunches. The dirt and gravel road ran straight into the building, allowing the trucks to drive in, dump their loads into the furnace, and drive on through. Just as the road reached the opening of the building, it was joined by another that wound up through the mounds of refuse. I had had the idea, and Rick had agreed, that it would be fun to race down that road straight at the workers while they were eating lunch and at the last moment turn off on the side road to the left; Jimmy would open the door and I would shove the watermelon out. If all went according to our plan, the watermelon would sail straight at the workmen, land just in front of them, burst, and scare hell out of everybody. Jimmy Casteen had grave doubts. Rick, as usual, was too enthusiastic, playing his part to exaggeration.

"You're going too fast," Jimmy yelled. "Slow down."

"Slow it down, Rick. You'll never make the turn," I said.

Rick ignored us both as he imagined himself driving the Indianapolis 500. He was hunched over the steering wheel, a determined look on his face, the accelerator pressed to the floor.

The workmen had watched with mounting interest as the car sped toward them, trailing great clouds of billowing dust.

"Turn," Jimmy hollered, "turn!" as we hurled past the place we were supposed to turn.

I released the watermelon. Jimmy dived to the floor and was muttering something I couldn't understand. I hoped it was a prayer. The car was almost in the building when Rick cut it hard to the left. We slid for a moment and then were scooting down the side road—backward. I braced for the inevitable. Rick, with a look of bewilderment, found it impossible to believe he was losing the Indianapolis 500. The rear fender snagged a pile of garbage, the car bounced once, landed on its side, and slid down the road, stopping a few feet from an enormous pit.

"Is everybody all right?" I asked.

"Yeah, I am. I'm okay," answered Rick.

"Jimmy, you okay?"

Jimmy was muttering something neither of us could make out. I climbed around the seat and found Jimmy lying on his side, eyes wide, holding the watermelon and muttering, "Where's the knife? What happened to the knife?"

"It's under your shoulder. You're lying on it," I told him.

"Oh, God, am I cut? Am I bleeding?"

"No. Now get out of the car. Come on."

We climbed out and I lied to the workmen about how the accelerator had hung, how Rick had tried in vain to stop the runaway car, how frightening it had all been. The workmen were very sympathetic and, with the aid of a garbage truck, helped right the overturned car. To everyone's surprise, the motor started. We pulled the crumpled fenders off the tires and found that it ran as well as ever.

Jimmy kept pacing back and forth mumbling to himself. The workmen thought he was crazy, that he had hit his head and should be taken to the hospital.

"Come on, Jimmy, get in. Let's go," I pleaded.

"I ain't getting in there," Jimmy shouted. "I'll walk home. You're crazy! Both of you. I could have been stabbed to death. Stabbed! In a car wreck. Do you *believe* that?" Jimmy Casteen walked off through the garbage, mumbling to himself.

Thinking back about it now, I wondered aloud, "Maybe Jimmy was right. Maybe we are a little crazy."

Rick shrugged.

We talked for a long time. I tried to explain what it was like to be paralyzed. Rick pretended to understand. We compared the experiences of our first year of college. We each lied a little. I told Rick that I did not plan to go back to Western Carolina, that I hoped to go to the University of Georgia. Rick was encouraging me to come to the University of North Carolina and room with him.

"I can't. Western is on the quarter system, and I have to transfer to a school on that system or I will lose too many credits," I was saying as Mom came back in.

"Well, old partner, I better be hitting the road. It's a long drive home."

"It was good to see you. Take it easy driving back."

Rick turned to Mom and winked. "That's a fine boy you got there. *A fine boy.* I don't know if I could—"

"Get outta here," I growled.

"See you later." He laughed as he closed the door behind him.

5

CURTIS RHINEHARDT placed one hand beneath my left knee; with the other he firmly grasped my heel and flexed my leg.

"Push," he demanded.

Sweat was running off my face and I could feel the veins in my neck bulging like taut wet ropes, and I strained to move. God, I wanted to move. I imagined my leg straightening with the speed and power it once had, my heel catching Rhinehardt just above the upper lip and driving his nose back into his head.

"Push. Come on, push, push, push," Rhinehardt snapped in a grating falsetto voice. "I get so tired of you people. If you must feel sorry for yourself, go ahead. But don't expect me to work miracles."

The words stung but I let them pass unanswered, as I did all of Rhinehardt's insults. For an hour each morning and each afternoon, we went through the routine of his flexing and extending my every muscle. We seldom spoke. I had disliked him on sight, and by now had come to despise him. For almost three weeks, Curtis Rhinehardt had belittled, baited, and harassed me. At first I thought the insults and exaggerated displays of disgust were being used as ploys to gain the maximum effort from me. But it soon became evident that they were something else altogether. Rhinehardt was simply a bully—a tyrant who practiced his tyranny on the physically helpless.

He was a small, effeminate man whose nervous, darting eyes were like little black beads set close together in a thin, pock-marked face. His yellowish-brown, cigarette-stained teeth protruded, stretching his lips in a perpetually taunting snarl.

Rhinehardt moved to my right leg and began to repeat the flexing procedure. "Let's at least try to stay awake, huh, Mr. Helms? That's not asking too much of you, now is it?"

The days and weeks in passing had been a kind of bleeding, a draining of energy. The exercises had not stemmed the gradual ebbing of muscle, the melting away of flesh. I was growing weaker each day, and each day brought with it less hope.

"Push," Rhinehardt chided.

It was near the end of the session and I was exhausted, spent, my breath coming in short puffs.

"Why, I do believe he's tired," he taunted, holding my left leg aloft with one finger beneath the heel. "Is that it? Is he tired?" he said, raising and lowering my leg effortlessly.

I eyed him impassively and waited.

With a chuckle he lowered my leg, flipped the sheet over it, and looked up at me with absolute disgust.

"Try something for me," I said.

"And what would that be? Walk on water?"

"No. When you go home tonight, lie down on your bed and tilt your head back, like me, so you don't see anything but the ceiling. Then try to move your ear. Don't wiggle your nose or raise your eyebrows, just make your ears move. And keep trying for a full hour. Give it everything you've got, don't think about anything else, make your ear move because you say it's going to move."

"Now, that would be rather foolish of me, wouldn't it? I would expect even you to know that the physical mechanism required to move one's ear simply does not exist," he said, moving to the side of the bed.

"I know. There's just no way to get a message out there, is there? Just like there's no way I can get one to my arms or legs. I just thought that if you tried, you might understand what I'm up against. You might understand what I'm trying to do and how hard it—"

Rhinehardt's arm shot out. He grabbed my face and squeezed hard, forcing my lips into an exaggerated pucker. Bending down slowly, he brought his face close, his mouth open in a downward grimace.

"How dare you," he hissed. "How dare you presume to know what I understand or don't understand. Why you—you insufferable—"

The muscles of my face tightened, pulling the flesh of my cheeks from his grasp and twisting my face into a feral mask of hatred and rage.

"Move it!" I said. "Move it or I'll tear your goddamn arm off." The words hissed out of me in a seething whisper.

My anger took him by surprise. He jerked his hand away and took a step back.

I had the advantage and now was the time to press it. In a street situation, this would be the time to hit him. Hit him hard and end it, but this wasn't the street.

"Who do you think you're talking to?" he sputtered in a high-pitched screech, trying to regain control of the situation.

"I know who I'm talking to, you son-of-a-bitch." I spat the words at him. "I know you. You didn't have the balls to take your lumps coming up, you couldn't cut it then, but you're hell now, aren't you. A real bad ass with old women and scared kids. Well, I ain't no old lady and I ain't no scared kid and I've had it with you, you sadistic little bastard."

"I don't have to listen to this," he sputtered, bringing his fists down against the outside of his legs in a gesture of frustration.

"No, you don't have to, but what you do have to do is come

in here and do your job and keep your fucking mouth shut. You got that? Keep your mouth shut. Because I'm going to get up from here one day! You know it and I know it. And if you ever say one more word to me than is absolutely necessary, do you know what I'm going to do? Huh? Do you? I'm gonna cancel your ride, fucker. I'm going to move your ears for you. Now get the hell out of here."

"Dr. McKinnon's gonna hear about this," he yelled over his shoulder.

When Mom came in a few minutes later, she took one look at me and shook her head. "I thought Mr. Rhinehardt was in a huff when he stormed by me."

"You mean he wasn't skipping down the hall?"

"He glared at me as if I were some kind of—some kind of insect."

"Well, don't worry about him. I think you could take him two out of three."

"I guess I knew it had to come, sooner or later, but I can't help feeling sorry for him."

"Sorry? For that—that—"

"Tom. Not just for him, but for people like him. Cruel, ineffectual little men whose only triumphs come wrapped in the misfortunes of others. Jackals snapping at ailing lions and in that moment believing themselves to be lions."

I looked up with surprise. "You been reading again?"

"Why?" She giggled. "Did you read that somewhere?"

"I don't know. Did you?"

"I don't know, but it sounded good."

"And it fit."

"At least the jackal part." She smiled. She didn't question me about what had happened; instead, she told me about her phone call home, about what my brother was doing, and who had asked about me.

She was telling me how my father had been unable to convince Mrs. Troxler, an old friend of the family, that I had not

54

suffered irrevocable brain damage, when Dr. McKinnon came into the room. He stood for a moment, looking at me as though he was having trouble deciding exactly what I was. He ran his tongue back and forth along the edge of his teeth and looked thoughtful.

"I've just spoken to Mr. Rhinehardt," he began. Then he paused and waited for me to defend my actions. When I didn't, he sighed and said, "I feel I must remind you that he is a member of my staff and due a certain amount of respect. I realize that his manner, at times, seems abrupt, but he is an excellent therapist and I hope nothing like this occurs again. We're all doing everything in our power to see to your well-being, and I would hope that you would appreciate these efforts."

"It's not that I don't appreciate it, Doc. I do," I said. "But if I were on my feet I wouldn't put up with Rhinehardt's abuse, and just because I'm flat on my back doesn't mean anything's changed. I thought it was time Rhinehardt realized that."

"I know that he can be exasperating, but he is a good therapist, technically, and there isn't any excuse for the way you talked to him," he said, looking sharply at me.

"Maybe he is good, technically, and I can use his help, but I'm going to walk out of here with or without him."

The sharpness in Dr. McKinnon's eyes gave way to a weary resolve. He exhaled tiredly. When he spoke, his voice was gentle. "That's brings us to another point. How long's it been? Thirty-seven, thirty-eight days, a little over five weeks; I think it's time you prepared yourself to accept the possibility that there may not be any more return. I feel that the sooner you can come to terms with that, the easier it will be."

I looked at him, not sure I heard correctly. "Prepare myself to accept the possibility? Doc, that just doesn't make sense. Do you go into surgery prepared to lose? How can anyone expect to win if he goes in prepared to lose? Can you see a guy going into a championship fight and saying, 'I hope to

55

win, but I'm prepared to lose'? No sir, it just doesn't work like that."

"We're not talking about sports."

"You bet we're not! But we're talking about a fight, and it's one I can't afford to lose. It won't be any easier to accept that loss today than it will be a year from now. What have I got to lose? If I accept it today, I'm stuck here for the rest of my life. So why not take my best shot? When I don't have anything left, then I'll accept it. What will it cost me? I got nothing else to do anyway."

"You have a limited amount of energy, and it's going to become even more limited," he explained. "In order for you to accomplish anything at all, it's going to be necessary to channel that energy. There's a hospital in Charlotte, a rehabilitation hospital that's set up to handle quadriplegics. They have facilities that we don't, and they specialize in this type of rehabilitative treatment. We'd like to send you down there just as soon as possible. I'd say in about four weeks, just as soon as the tongs come out."

This was something new. I knew I was getting weaker, but I hadn't realized that my energy and thus my concentration were running out.

"Doc, what are my chances of moving again?"

"I'd say there's still a possibility of some return to the shoulders and upper arms. You'd be surprised—"

"What are the odds of my walking again?"

"I don't make odds, Mr. Helms. It's my medical opinion that you won't. If you insist on odds, I'll have to refer you to a bookmaker."

"How many patients in my condition would you have to have before one walked out? One out of a hundred? A thousand?"

Dr. McKinnon looked down at the floor, frowning.

"Ten thousand? One out of ten thousand?" I was pushing.

He looked up wearily, shaking his head slowly. "I'm afraid

you'll have to talk to a theologian to get your odds. How often do miracles occur? One in a thousand? Ten thousand? It's not my intent to be cruel, Mr. Helms. It's just that once you accept the fact that this is the way it's going to be, you can begin to adjust your goals. Once you're in Charlotte, you can channel your energies toward learning to use what you have with the aids available to you. There are some remarkable devices on the market today. I think you'll be surprised at what you'll be able to accomplish."

"Turning on the TV by mashing a button with my chin? That sort of thing?" I growled.

"Among other things, yes," he continued. "They're coming out with more sophisticated things every day."

I stared at him with disgust. I could feel the corners of my mouth turning down as if I had suddenly encountered something repugnant.

"Well, there will be time to discuss it later," he said as he turned and walked out of the room.

I stared at the ceiling and felt the muscles of my jaw tighten into knots. "It's my medical opinion that you won't." The words kept repeating themselves. Well, his medical opinion was wrong. I didn't give a damn about his opinion anyway, it was his facts that worried me most. My energy was going to become more limited, and that meant I would soon have trouble concentrating for long periods of time. I had to be able to concentrate. I had to be able to hold a single thought, and hold it for hours.

I didn't see Mom standing there until she touched my forehead. She had one hand on my arm and was brushing something imaginary from my forehead. It was the only gesture of affection she could make. She looked down with a bittersweet smile, and I knew she was searching for something to say. It was then that I realized how desperately helpless she must feel. At least I had that toe. At least I could try. But she could do absolutely nothing.

I smiled, slowly and devilishly. "Got ya in a bind, haven't they, old girl?"

She was thirty-six years old and trim as a schoolgirl. She had been mistaken for my sister so often that I had begun calling her "old girl" as a joke.

"A bind?" she asked, looking puzzled.

"Yes, you want to be encouraging but you don't want to encourage any false hope, right?"

"Wrong. Sometimes I wonder about you," she mused. "Maybe Mrs. Troxler is right. Maybe there is brain damage." She leaned down and kissed me on the forehead.

I scowled at her. I hated that and she knew it.

She smiled down triumphantly. Then her eyes grew soft, and when she spoke, her voice was low and gentle and serious. "Tom, when you were born I was eighteen years old—a child. We grew up together. Sometimes I didn't know who was parent and who was child, and sometimes I think you were never a child at all. Maybe it's because you were my firstborn, or maybe all mothers feel this way, but I believe in you. I don't think there's anything you can't do if you want it bad enough. If you say you're going to walk, I believe it, and I'll go on believing it as long as you do."

"Well, it looks like we're up against some pretty long odds."

She smiled. "Didn't you tell me about that special blue sky of yours?"

"Yes, and the reason I told you was so you wouldn't worry."

"Who's worried? Do I look worried?"

I eyed her carefully. "No. No, you don't."

She looked at me for a long time, her smile sly and mysterious, as if she saw something deep in me that made her proud. Then she said, "There is one thing."

"What?"

"I wish you would try to let some of the emotion out—"

"Aw, Mom, don't start that now."

"I just don't think it's good—"

58

"I let some out. I let it out on Rhinehardt, and look where that got us."

"That's anger. That's all you've shown. That's what worries Dr. McKinnon, and that's what worries me."

"I thought you weren't worried."

"I'm worried! I'm worried!" she exclaimed in exasperation.

I smiled.

She sat down and began reading.

I had tried to get it out. Dr. McKinnon had expressed his concern about my apparently stoic attitude, my lack of emotional response, and she had wrung from me a promise to try, in the privacy of night, to "get it all out," to yell or scream or cry. I had kept the promise. In the darkness of the predawn hours, I had indulged myself with self-pity and came close to tears several times. But each time I did, I would suddenly see the hospital as a Norman Rockwell painting I remembered. He had painted an apartment house with the front wall removed so the occupants of the various apartments could be seen pursuing their various lives. Each time tears threatened, I found myself standing outside, looking at the hospital with its front wall removed, exposing its imagined patients. Above me I saw an old man at the end of his life, sad and confused because life's promise had not been kept, feeling an empty despair, a vague sense of something missed as he looked back over his life. Beside me a young mother tried to reconcile the imagined, hoped-for emotions she had thought would accompany the birth of her first child with the tragically real horror of the pitifully twisted, deformed infant. Below me a young man sat holding his wife's hand, watching a lifetime of dreams, plans, hopes, and the future dying with her. In the middle of it all, I saw myself as the only one with any hope, lying in the darkness of my room trying to cry. I felt only disgust and contempt for my futile effort at tears. I had no tears for myself. I would never have, not as long as there was hope, and if that failed, there would always be the anger.

For the next two weeks I intensified my efforts, straining every fiber of my being, concentrating so completely on moving that one toe that I began to lose contact with my surroundings. I was having trouble remembering nurses' names, had to ask if it was day or night. Once I even alarmed Mom by squinting at her fiercely for endless seconds before recognizing her. I was retreating deeper and deeper into myself where an awesome devastating battle raged. The exercises continued but did not slow the wasting away of muscle and flesh. Rhinehardt continued his twice daily visits but never looked me in the eye and never spoke other than to mumble an occasional "push" or "pull."

My father came up for the weekend and brought Wayne for the first time. Mom had insisted that I "take the weekend off" so as not to alarm my brother. The rest and their visit lightened my mood and relieved the pressure that had been building. At my prodding, Mom had consented to get away from the hospital for a while. They had just left for an outing in the mountains when the door opened.

"Well, hard leg," Rick said, "where is everybody?"

"Out," I said.

"In that case, while they're off the premises," he intoned solemnly, "I wonder if I might interest you in what is considered among connoisseurs to be the finest collection of pornographic literature in existence today. A veritable gold mine, a godsend, if you will." Pulling an imaginary volume from a make-believe coat, he waved it aloft in the manner of a stump preacher, intoxicated by his own rhetoric. "My friend, never, I say never, has man achieved such soaring heights in his literary endeavors. Contained herein are sights never before seen by man, feats never before performed by mortal man. Guaranteed to stimulate, titillate, arouse you to passions henceforth limited to those that dwell upon Olympus. And I am prepared, my friend, to place in your hot little hands this masterpiece,

60

for the trifling sum of five dollars. Think of it, my boy—for five scruffy, measly, insignificant little greenbacks, paradise is yours."

"Is that any way to come into a sick person's room?"

"Sick! Sick, you say! Why son, sick is what this book is all about. Only the mind of a sick human being could fully appreciate this cornucopia of erotic delights."

"I'm lying here on death's doorstep and you come in here acting like that," I said, suppressing a smile.

"Doorstep? Doorstep?" he repeated thoughtfully. Wetting his finger, he leafed through the imaginary book. "Ah, yes, doorstep. Here we are, chapter three, positions forty-six and one hundred and seven as demonstrated—now get this—on a doorstep. Yes sir, something for everyone." We both roared with laughter.

Then I could see it in his eyes. It was only there for a moment, like a shadow moving across his face, but it was the reason I wouldn't look into a mirror. I was losing weight rapidly. What had once been powerfully muscled arms were thin pipe stems lying useless at my side, and I could feel the skin drawing tight across my cheekbones. My hair was growing back darker, having been spared the bleaching effects of the elements, and it would serve to accentuate the hospital pallor of my face.

Rick shook off his momentary melancholy, and a slow smile crawled across his face as he jerked his thumb over his shoulder toward the door and said in a whisper, "Hey, man, who's that nurse with the legs?"

I looked at him unbelievingly.

"You know. The one with short brown hair and a great set of legs. I mean legs like I like."

"Sometimes I wonder how you find your way home."

"What? You don't think she has great legs?"

"How the hell would I know? All I can see is faces when I'm on my back and feet when I'm on my stomach. I don't have any idea what's in between."

"Oh. Okay, guess who's home."

"I don't know."

"Rene Crawford. She's been dancing all over Europe with some group out of New York. Talk about a set of legs. I took her out Tuesday night and—"

"I don't wanna hear about it."

"Shit. You're sicker than I thought."

"No, it's not that. I just don't want to get that on my mind. All I do is lie here and think. I don't sleep very much and—damn, ole Rene does have a fine set of walkers on her, doesn't she?"

"You don't know the half of it, listen—"

"I don't want to hear it."

"Okay, okay. I got a message from Herb."

"Herb Brockman?"

"Yeah. We were all a little soused the other night and he said to ask you what great truth you've realized."

"Huh?"

"Well, according to Herb, when you come close to dying your whole life flashes in front of you and you realize some profound truth."

"Where the hell did he get that idea?"

"Well"—he started laughing—"it seems that when Herb was about fifteen his old man walked in on him and caught him whippin' off."

"And his whole life flashed in front of him?"

"Yeah." He laughed. "Said he thought he was going to have a heart attack and his whole damn life flashed in front of him."

"What," I finally got out through the laughter, "was his great truth?"

"He said he had a vision that he hasn't figured out to this day. Won't tell anybody what it was."

We were quiet for a while. Then Rick asked seriously, "Did your life flash before you? I mean, I've heard of that happening with people who almost drown."

"No, my life didn't flash before me and I didn't realize anything profound," I told him. "But I do think I know what's important to me now."

"What?"

"Look, you know the feeling when you've been bangin' some nice young thing and you're lying there staring at the ceiling, wondering what to say, wishing she would disappear and that empty feeling you have like something that ought to be there wasn't? That feeling of something missing?"

"Do I ever."

"Well, what do you think it is? What's missing?"

"How the hell would I know?"

"Well, I know, and I should have known that weekend up at Women's College in Greensboro when I spent the whole, entire weekend in the sack in a motel. And when I took her back to the dorm and started—"

"You didn't tell me about that."

"I'm telling you now."

"Who was she? Becky?"

"No."

"Joyce?"

"No."

"It was Becky, wasn't it?"

"No, it was not Becky. It wasn't anybody you know. Now, are you going to let me get on with it or not?"

"Okay, all right." He pouted.

"Well, anyway, I was completely wrung out. I mean if Marilyn Monroe had jumped in the car naked and put a gun to my head I couldn't have gotten it up."

"It was Becky all right," he said with a knowing smile.

I took a deep breath and exhaled loudly. "Would you get off that. Now, as I was saying, I was wiped out and I was riding along and I suddenly felt horny. No way, not after that weekend. It had to be something else. An emotional horniness, maybe. I mean it couldn't have been physical, I didn't have anything physical left. Right?"

"Right," he agreed.

"Okay, so if it wasn't physical, all the bodies in the world couldn't have satisfied it. It wouldn't make a damn how good-looking she was. So what it boils down to is loving somebody."

Rick furrowed his brow in thought.

"I mean, there I was riding along all content and satisfied, and I just wanted to turn to somebody I cared about and say, "Ain't the world a beautiful place to be?" I was feeling good, I didn't want to screw anybody, I wanted to love somebody. And that's what it's all about—loving somebody."

"Then what you're trying to say is we feel empty because we don't love 'em. And you think that's what's missing?"

"That's right. Once you've got ol' Leroy quieted down, the real need pops up. The need to love somebody, and because you don't love that body lying beside you, you get that feeling of something missing. And it's not just in ballin' either, it's true in everything. You go ahead and get rich and famous, and one day you'll look around and something's wrong, it's not like it ought to be, something's missing and you got an empty feeling deep in your gut."

"You really think it'll be like that?"

"Damn right I do. How many famous people at the top of their careers—I mean people that have made it big, movie stars, sports figures, painters, authors, that sort—have you read about that knocked themselves off, and it came out later that they were all messed up because nobody loved 'em or they couldn't find anybody they could love?"

"A bunch."

"Damn right, a bunch. Who was that king that abdicated so he could marry the girl he loved?"

"Henry the Eighth?"

"No, hell no, not Henry the Eighth." I laughed. "It was Charles or Edward the something or other—anyway, whoever he was, he had the right idea. He knew life wasn't going to be worth a damn without her, even if he was a king. Being king ain't what it's all about, and everybody knows it. They know it without even knowing they know. It's built in, back in the back of your brain somewhere, and everybody's running around looking for it and not knowing exactly what it is they're looking for. But knowing just the same that if they don't find it they won't ever be whole."

"I think I see what you're drivin' at, Amos, and now that I think about it, you're probably right, but I'll just be damned if I plan to tell that to Herb."

"Well, make up something to tell him."

The door opened and a gruff, grizzled man walked into the room. His outdated suit was hopelessly rumpled, as though he had slept in it and had come directly from his bed without bothering to shave or comb his oily, matted hair. He ran a dirty, callused hand across the stubble on his chin, making a rasping sound, and leveled his gaze on me. "You been saved?" he asked.

"I'm Jewish," I said. Rick's mouth fell open. He looked from me to the man to see if he would challenge it.

The man looked bored and sighed tiredly, like he was going to have to explain something that no one seemed to understand. "Don't make no difference. Lord don't care what denomination a man is, as long as he accepts Christ as his savior."

I just looked at him for a moment. "Well, to tell you the truth, this is Rabbi Rubenstein"—I cut my eyes toward Rick—"and we were right in the middle of confession."

Rick fought back the grin that threatened his serious composure. The man studied him for a moment, nodded his head tiredly, and started for the door. "Well, I won't keep you, Brother."

"Who was that?" Rick asked, once he was gone.

"I don't know. Probably some logger that got tired of cutting trees and took up preaching. The place is crawling with 'em. Listen, if anybody around here asks you if you been saved, you better say yes. Because if you don't, you're in for the prayin' of your life."

"Yeah?" He grinned.

"Yeah. They come in here all the time, four and five a day, and ask if they can pray for me. What can I say? You can't tell somebody they can't pray for you. So I say okay. I been prayed over more than anybody in history."

"You need it more than anybody in history."

"Listen, you just don't know," I told him. "There was one guy found out I hadn't been saved and he launched into prayer to beat the band. I mean, he really got worked up, kept asking if I felt the spirit. I didn't know what the hell to say. I was going to fake it. I've never seen anybody with the spirit, but I've heard that they jump around and shake and holler and carry on something awful. But I couldn't figure any way to pull that off."

"What'd you do?"

"I didn't do anything. I just kept telling him I didn't feel anything. It was real embarrassing. He was working so hard waving that Bible, and big tears were rollin' down his face. Finally I let fly with 'hallelujah' as loud as I could and that seemed to satisfy him. He calmed down and said, 'Ain't it a glorious feeling to be saved?' and I said it sure was and he left."

We talked for a while then about revival meetings and being saved, and wondered what the girls that went to them were like. We were still talking when my supper tray came. Rick stood up to leave. "Somebody coming to feed you that?"

"Yeah. Mom'll be back before long."

"Well, ol' pardner, I'll be seeing you. You'll probably be in Charlotte by the time I get loose again. This working seven days a week is for the damn birds."

He left and the room screamed, the silence was so loud. It waited there in the silence, dark, oppressive, and inescapable. For precious seconds I clung to that part of the world Rick had brought with him. Then I faced it. My mood darkened and I felt the aching press of weight. "You're going to move, you stubborn bastard. You're going to move."

The next afternoon Mom was sitting by my bed reading. I had been lost in concentration for hours when it happened. A wild, joyous, panicky eagerness raced through me. It moved! *The toe moved.* It wasn't anything I could feel as much as it was something I knew. It moved. I wanted to yell and holler and laugh and cry. I had to stop. I had to hold back the swelling excitement. I had to think. Had it really moved? I hadn't actually felt it. Maybe it hadn't moved at all. I reached out straining to feel, groping with dead nerves to feel, striving with useless muscles to feel, taxing my ears for the slightest sound of movement. Nothing. I could feel nothing. I could hear nothing above the pounding roar of my blood. Yet it moved. I *knew* it had moved. "Mom," I whispered, fighting back the tremors of ebullition that swept through me, "Mom, look at my foot a minute. My right foot." I was working feverishly as she picked up the sheet and looked down.

"Okay. I'm looking," she said.

"You don't see it?"

"See what, hon?"

"Are you looking at my right foot?" I snapped. "The big toe on my right foot?"

"Yes."

"And it's not moving?"

"No," she said, bending down closer. "I can't see it."

"You can't see it!" I yelled. "You gotta see it. It's moving, I tell you. You're not lookin'! *Look!*" I poured all of my strength, every last bit of energy, every ounce of desire into one last massive effort.

She looked up with sad, helpless eyes. "I'm sorry, son. It's just not moving."

I exploded. "I tell you, it's moving! I beat it! I beat it! It's moving. I know it's moving," I screamed.

For the first time Mom caught a glimpse of the awesome forces that were raging within me, and it frightened her. "Wait a second," she said. "Maybe . . . maybe it is moving, just a—"

"Don't do that, Momma. Don't lie to me. If it's not moving, for God's sake, don't lie to me."

"I'm sorry . . . I'm . . . you just wanted it to move so bad," she said. Dropping the sheet over the motionless foot, she moved to the side of the bed and reached out for my arm. She stopped suddenly, staring, the breath caught in her throat. "Tom," she said softly, "try it again."

I looked up at her and saw the desperate, pleading expression.

"Just do it, Tom. Try."

The muscles of my face tightened, I clenched my teeth grimly, pushed through a smothering exhaustion, and tried with all that was left in me to move a single toe.

Mom looked down at me, smiling through a rush of tears. "It's not your toe, it's your thumb. You're moving your thumb."

I stared at her in utter disbelief. "My *thumb?* I'm moving my thumb? All this time . . . all this time . . . and it's my thumb?" She nodded, unable to find her voice because of the tears. I tried to hold it back but I couldn't. It started small, down in my throat, little jerking chuckles that grew and spread and swelled until the laughter rolled out of me in waves. Waves that filled the room and crashed against the walls. Great billowing gales of laughter roaring up out of me, bringing with it long weeks of agonizing pain and anger, endless nights of bitter loneliness and frustration and hate—laughter that was a release, an escape, laughter that tore down the imprisoning walls of paralysis. Laughter rang out of me like a song. I laughed at myself, at my toe, at Rhinehardt, at Dr. McKinnon. I laughed at my mother trying to lie, and at my thumb, that poor neglected, forgotten champion of a thumb. I laughed at it all.

Two days later I moved my toe and continued moving it day and night, awake or asleep. My progress was measured daily, hourly, but it was mostly sensation, the return of feeling. The wasted, atrophied muscles were going to have to be rebuilt, retrained. The simplest physical task required all my straining effort and concentration and willpower. Once I looked up triumphantly at Mom after touching my thumb and index finger. The effort had taken three days. Three days of concentration, of straining and sweating and cursing. And with the completion of that simple act, I joined, in spirit, that select brotherhood of men who know the exhilaration, the intoxicating headiness of conquest, of pushing through age-old barriers to stand alone atop unscaled mountains.

By the time Dr. McKinnon was ready to remove the tongs, I had full return of sensation. I was able, with great effort, to wiggle all my fingers and toes and to bend, slightly, my knees and elbows.

6

THE huge black orderly took his time pushing the stretcher down the hall toward the gym, and that suited me. I was in no hurry to get there. I pushed my chin out as far as I could and moved it around; it didn't help, so I shifted it to the left, saw that wasn't going to work, then tried moving it to the right. The steel and leather brace did not fit properly. It cut my chin and held my head crooked, cocked to one side. The walking shorts and sport shirt I was required to wear were uncomfortable and, after ten weeks of lying naked beneath a sheet, seemed to bind and restrict my limited movement. I hiked one shoulder, trying to correct the position of my head, and the chin cup cut deeper into my raw, tender jaw, adding to an already black mood.

Dr. McKinnon had referred me to Dr. Robert Walters, and the entire morning had been devoted to a long examination, during which I had been brought to a sitting position for the first time, allowing me to see the terrible effects of the previous weeks. I had stared in mute shock at my pitifully thin arms and legs. It was a stranger's body, one whose shape and lines were new and unfamiliar to me. I had lost forty-two pounds, and as I surveyed the remains of a once powerful body, I felt sick, physically and emotionally sick.

The morning had left me despondent and strangely tired. It was not the horror of witnessing the physical devastation so much as it was the sudden realization of what lay ahead. It was not going to be a simple matter of getting into shape again. I would have to rebuild my entire body and that would take time, a lot of time. I watched the ceiling pass slowly overhead as the orderly made his way down the long hall, and I told myself that at least I wasn't as bad off as Hal Boman. Bo, as he preferred to be called, was one of my two new roommates. He was a twenty-six-year-old engineer who had broken his neck diving into shallow water two years earlier. He reminded me of pictures I had seen of Dachau. Bo was a living skeleton; every bone in his body was visible. He was in the hospital for surgery on pressure sores he had acquired due to neglect by the staff of the nursing home where he lived. He had been sent to the home after a year of therapy, when it was determined that no further progress could be expected.

My other roommate was Glen Teeter. Although I had arrived the previous evening, I had not yet seen him. Glen Teeter never talked to anybody and insisted on keeping his head covered. According to Bo, Glen was eighteen years old and had broken his neck in an automobile six months earlier. Bo explained that it was hospital policy to put patients with similar problems together in the hope that they would help each other adjust. There were no private rooms because most patients were long-term, and being alone could just increase the feelings of depression and self-pity. He told me that the fourth bed in our room would probably remain empty, unless the hospital became crowded, until another male patient with a broken neck arrived.

The orderly parked the stretcher in the corner of the gym and left. I dreaded what was to come. I had spent the previous evening talking with Bo and had learned that my therapist was to be Don Stirewalt. Bo did not try to conceal his hatred for Stirewalt. He told me that he was a huge brute from somewhere in Pennsylvania who enjoyed pushing people around, and he advised me not to let Stirewalt get the upper hand or life would be miserable for me. Stirewalt would try, according to Bo, to break my spirit on the first meeting, and from there on he would insist on doing exercises that were impossible and would not lead to walking or anything else. "Let him know from the start that you're not going to do one damned thing. Nobody ever gets well anyway, so why go through all that. He'll get mad and cuss like a sailor, but he'll do that anyway. If you don't, he'll stay on your back, always pushing and harassing hell out of you," Bo had said. I was in no mood to be pushed or harassed. I wanted to be left alone. I needed time to adjust to the things I had seen during the examination, time to prepare myself for the long painful struggle that lay ahead, time to decide how best to deal with Stirewalt. I worked my chin around in a futile effort to escape the pressure and ease the pain.

"Helms?" the man asked.

"Yes," I said, looking up. I knew immediately who the man was, even though he was younger than I had expected him to be. He was in his early thirties, broadly built, and heavy but not fat. He wore dark blue pants and a white shirt that stretched tight over massive shoulders. The short sleeves of his shirt were held down tight on his upper arms by powerful, bulging muscles. His massive, leonine head seemed almost too small for the thick, muscular neck that supported it. His face, squared by a granite jaw, was pale and close-shaven but bore a perpetual shadow from the blue-black stubble of his thick beard. The thick horn-rimmed glasses he wore magnified his heavy, protruding brown eyes, giving him the petulant look of a mischievous child. He ran his short, stubby fingers through a shock of wild black hair and pushed it carelessly to one side of his forehead. His deep bass voice rumbled up through a barrel chest.

72

"I'm Don Stirewalt," he said. Looking at the ill-fitting brace, he shook his massive head and exhaled in exasperation. "Let me see if I can help you with that." He began gently making adjustments on the brace, explaining to me that the two steel posts supporting the chin cup varied in length by more than an inch. "Who the hell set this rig up?"

"The therapist in Asheville," I told him.

"Well, he sure screwed it up," he growled. "I don't think he knew what the hell he was doing."

"Oh, I think he knew," I said. "I think he knew exactly what he was doing."

Stirewalt looked at me, puzzled, and waited expectantly. When I offered no further comment, he turned silently back to working on the brace. My head slowly lost its tilt and rested normally, cupped by the brace. He wedged a chubby finger between the cup and my chin and pressed down. "Jesus," he growled, "did you know you're bleeding?" He walked off across the gym cursing under his breath. When he returned he had a piece of foam rubber which he carefully molded to fit the cup. "That should feel a little better," he said.

For the next hour he conducted a muscle test, carefully charting the strength and range of every muscle, explaining what exercises would be necessary to strengthen them. Completing the test, he lay his clipboard to one side. "Before we can really get into anything more than mat exercises, you're going to have to spend some time on the tilt table," he said, nodding toward a long padded table covered in red vinyl with straps hanging loosely from its sides.

I frowned. "Why?"

"That allows us to bring you to a standing position slowly. A few degrees each day. You've been lying flat so long that if we didn't do that, you'd get sick and black out every time you tried to stand or sit."

"I don't think I'll have to do that," I said irritably. "I sat up this morning and I didn't black out. I felt a little dizzy at first, but it passed. Look, I'm in a hurry. I just don't have time to lie around on some table for a couple of days."

"All right, if you think you can tolerate it." He smiled knowingly. "We might as well get started right now. First of all, we're going to have to loosen you up, going to have to do some stretching." Walking to the foot of the stretcher, he picked up my foot and placed the heel of it on his broad shoulder. His huge hand swallowed my knee as he pressed it into a locked position. I felt the tendons in the back of my leg tighten. He stared speculatively at me for a moment, then rolled his shoulder forward, raising the angle of my leg, tightening the tendons. I flinched at the sudden surge of pain. Grinning wryly at me, Stirewalt took a step forward and studied me critically. I clenched my teeth against the growing pain, but did not take my eyes from Stirewalt's. The back of my leg was stretched so tight the tendons felt like steel cables, stinging and burning and singing with a hot, pulsing current. I saw the arrogant challenge in Stirewalt's eyes as he took another step. The knotted muscles of my jaw quivered as I returned his cold probing stare. We stared at each other for long seconds before he took another step, tightening the straining, aching tendons, increasing the hot flowing pain. He eyed me steadily, silently, without moving. I felt a warm sticky fluid oozing behind my knee. It was a senseless, brutal contest that had to stop. I choked back the moan that rose in my throat and glared fiercely at him as he took yet another unhurried step. I felt the sickening, burning sting of something tearing deep in my leg. The tendons were going to pull away from the bone if this did not stop. I wanted to scream but I held Stirewalt's gaze steady and level. I knew he would ease off if I asked him, but I would not ask him. I would not show him my pain. I would not break as Bo had broken. Stirewalt leaned his weight into the burning, resisting tendons and hung there, resting his great bulk against the screaming protest of muscle and bone, and continued to eye me unblinkingly. Black dots peppered my vision, swimming and dancing crazily before a hazy, blurring image of Stirewalt. I blinked away the milky haze and doggedly met his cold analytical stare, held it, returned it, and watched it change to one of mounting surprise and respect as he gradually eased the pressure on my leg.

I sighed with relief as my leg was slowly lowered to the stretcher. The sharp burning pain immediately subsided, replaced by a dull, throbbing ache. He looked at me curiously for a moment before turning and walking out of the gym. When he returned he stood silently folding a washcloth. I eyed him apprehensively. Impassively, without warning, he shoved the cloth into my mouth. The cold resolve deserted me as I vehemently spit the cloth out with a blistering stream of obscenities.

Stirewalt chuckled as he picked up the cloth. "You're a real hard nose, aren't you?"

"No, I'm not a hard nose," I said in a voice quavering with anger, "but I'm gonna walk again, by God. And if I have to go over every goddamn doctor and therapist in the whole fuckin' state, then that's what I'll do. But what I'm not gonna do is play your sick little game. I'm not gonna—"

"Whoa, hold on," he said. "You think that was a game? You think I enjoyed that little exercise? You think I enjoyed hurting you?"

I stared at him mutely, my eyes fixed, unwavering, accusing.

He was no longer amused by the situation. His expression was one of pained bewilderment. "My God! That is what you think," he said incredulously. "Why? What possible reason could I have?"

"I don't know why. Pulling wings off butterflies, I guess," I snapped. "I don't know."

"Pulling wings off . . ." His voice trailed off and he shook his massive head in disbelief. He looked down at me thoughtfully for a moment, then frowned. "You didn't understand what I was doing with this?" he said, holding the washcloth.

I looked up at him cautiously, perplexed.

"No, of course, you didn't," he said, disgusted with himself.

"I'm sorry. I can imagine what you must have thought." He laughed. "It's just that we've got a lot more to do and the way you were gritting your teeth, you were going to end up breaking one or ruining 'em all. And since I don't have a bullet, I thought you could bite on this."

"Well, why didn't you say so?"

"I don't know." He shrugged. "I guess I was busy watching your reactions and thinking ahead." He paused. "Look, there are two ways to go about this stretching; slow and easy, letting up before the pain gets too bad, but that takes weeks, sometimes months. Or, if you can stand the pain, we can continue the way we've started and cut it to days—a week or so. So far, we've done one leg one time. We're going to have to do both legs, both ankles, and your shoulders—twice a day, every day. Now, are you still in a hurry?"

"I'm still in a hurry," I said.

"Okay, but before we start I want you to understand something. I'm in just as big a hurry as you, and once we start I'm not going to let up," he said sternly. "I'm going to work you until you drop and then I'm going to work you some more. You're not going to *walk* out of here, you're going to run. You're going to be dancing up and down these halls before I'm through with you. I've waited for somebody like you all of my professional life, and now that I've got you—I'm going to push you all the way. You start dragging your ass, and I'm going to start chewing your ass."

I looked at him questioningly.

"Every quad I've ever worked with," he explained, "has asked me if I've ever seen anybody walk away from it. And every time I've had to say no. I've had to say no and stand there and watch something die in them, something in their eyes. It doesn't happen all at once, but that's when it begins. It's like a light in them was going out, getting dimmer and weaker, until finally their eyes are dull and smoky, and there's nothing left inside." He stood there silent, lost in the pain of remembering. I looked with surprise at a familiar anguish, a bitter sadness reflected in his broad face. He stared down blankly at me for a moment, without seeing me. Then he blinked his eyes quickly, as though to get back to some reality. "Did you notice Boman's eyes? He's dead. Inside he's dead. He could never have walked again, but if I could have gotten him to try, if I could have held out the hope . . ." He paused, searching for the words. "He should be able to *feed* himself, to scratch his nose when it itches, to read a book, maybe even write a letter or paint a picture. He should be able to light his own cigarettes, comb his hair, brush his teeth. He shouldn't have to call a nurse every time he wants the channel changed on the TV or needs a drink of water. He shouldn't have had to lie in that goddamn nursing home and rot while he waited for some dried-up old bitch to answer his buzzer. He told me once that he had looked forward to a TV program for over a month—that was a big thing for him, to actually look forward to something—he couldn't get them to come turn on the TV until the program was almost over." Stirewalt shook his head in bitter disgust. "He should be able to do a hundred small things that would make that living death more bearable. And he could have, if I'd been able to get him to make the effort. But he would have had to bust his ass to do it. He would have had to sweat and bleed and work and hurt day after day after day, for a hell of a long time. And for what? To comb his hair? To turn on a TV? It just wasn't worth the pain and the frustration. But, by God, if he had thought he had a chance of beating it, a chance of walking out of here, he would have made the effort."

"Is it too late now?" I asked, looking at him and seeing him for the first time.

"For Boman? Yes. The muscles are too atrophied," he said grimly, brushing at the washcloth with the back of his hand. Then he looked thoughtfully at me, his eyes glinting slyly with secret amusement. "You know it's a miracle that you're alive," he said.

"I know."

"I'm not going to see any more patients with their necks broken as bad as yours—as high as yours. They just don't live." He smiled cunningly. "I'm not only going to be able to tell them I've seen somebody beat it, I'm going to be able to tell them I've seen someone in worse shape than them dancing down the halls."

"Not if you stand there running your mouth all day you're not."

He laughed. I opened my mouth and he placed the folded washcloth between my teeth.

By the end of the week the washcloth was in shreds and I was in a wheelchair. I was sitting at one end of the gym trying, with Stirewalt's help, to lift my foot off the floor. Neither of us expected me to do it. The attempt was an exercise designed to strengthen the thighs. I was absently following his instructions looking beyond him to the far end of the gym where they had strapped Glen Teeter to the red tilt table. An aide was methodically turning a crank in the heavy base of the table and Glen was slowly coming into view. When he reached a forty-five-degree angle, the aide stopped and checked the straps before going off to another patient. It was the first time I had seen Glen other than an occasional glance back in our room. He was dressed in the standard sport shirt and walking shorts. He was short and as wasted as Bo. The nose was too big for his face and the skin was stretched tight and shiny across a knot in the middle of it. His weak-chinned, pimply face was cupped by a mass of shaggy blond curls. He stared out uninterestedly through dull, lifeless eyes and chewed rhythmically on a wad of chewing gum.

"How'd you get this scar?" Stirewalt asked.

"Huh?" I grunted, my attention still on Glen.

"The scar on your knee," he said. "How'd you get it?"

"Oh. My old man threw me out of a truck once."

"Your father threw you out of a truck?"

78

"Well, he didn't exactly throw me out, but he didn't do a whole lot to keep me in," I said, looking back at Glen.

Stirewalt looked up from his kneeling position with a puzzled frown knotting his busy eyebrows together. "Lift," he said, and waited as I flexed the muscles in my thigh. "Well? You going to tell me about it or not?"

I stared across the gym at Glen for a moment, then looked down at Stirewalt. "My old man bought a rickety-ass ol' panel truck one time just to knock around in—you know—for huntin' and fishin' and stuff, and it only had one seat in it. I had to sit on a box. We were goin' huntin' one day, and he told me to close my door—it hadn't latched or something. I must have been about fifteen at the time, and I wasn't paying any attention to the road or anything. So just as I opened the door he went around a sharp curve, the door flew open, and me and the box and everything else went flyin' out. Well, I grabbed the top of the door just as the box fell out from under me and started yelling for him to stop the truck. He kept right on driving. I was out there swinging on that door, yelling to beat the damn band, and he kept on driving. My feet were scraping the pavement and starting to hurt something awful so I let go—fell flat on my face and ended up in a drainage ditch full of water."

"Why didn't he stop?" Stirewalt asked.

"That's what I wanted to know. I figured he was trying to teach me a lesson or something. He was always saying I didn't pay attention to half of what I was supposed to. And I guess if I'd been paying attention, I wouldn't have opened that door just before we went into a curve. But I thought that was a pretty dumb-ass way to teach me anything, and that's just about as close as I ever came to punching my old man."

"Really pissed you off, did he?"

"Yeah, and I think he knew it too, because when I climbed up out of that ditch, he was running back down the road toward me but as soon as he saw my face he stopped, started backing up and explaining. Said he was trying to slow down gradually. Said he was afraid that if he stopped suddenly it would sling me off or something."

Stirewalt laughed. "Lift up, hard. That's it. Again."

I strained to raise my foot. "When we got home he made me tell Mom I fell in a creek, so she wouldn't worry the next time we went out in the truck."

"Lift."

"She said anybody that went around falling in creeks didn't have sense enough to handle a gun and she took my rifle away." I laughed. "Ain't that hell?"

Stirewalt laughed and sat back on the floor. "Relax a minute. Take a break." He laughed and shook his head. "You know, something like that happened with me and my old man once."

"Yeah?"

"We were on vacation and we were out on a pier fishing. I was sitting on the rail and my father spun around suddenly and knocked me off. I damn near drowned. He said he forgot I was sitting there."

"Did he make you lie about it when you got home?"

"No siree. I hated fishing, so when we got home I went straight to Mom and told her Pop had knocked me off the pier and I was lucky to be alive because the water was lousy with sharks. Man, did she chew his ass out."

"I'll bet he *loved* you for that." I laughed. I glanced back at Glen just as his eyes rolled back and his head lolled about dropping to one side. "Glen's passed out," I said excitedly.

Stirewalt shifted his weight around and looked in Glen's direction. He was on his feet instantly, racing across the gym. "You son-of-a-bitch," he screamed as he slammed his huge fist into the table inches from Glen's face. The force of the blow jarred the heavy table, shoving it back against the wall. Glen's eyes sprang open wide, staring in shock at the outraged Stirewalt. "You lousy little bastard, don't you ever pull a stunt like that again. You got me? I'll ship you out of here so fast you *will* pass out."

The ticking of the wall clock thundered through the silence that hung over the gym. Stirewalt, suddenly aware of the silence and the startled stares of the patients, lowered his voice to an angry whisper. "Look at that," he said, pointing to a four-year-old girl in full leg braces. "She's got more guts than you, more courage than you. She doesn't know the meaning of self-pity, but you could teach her, you could tell all about it, couldn't you?"

"Can I go back to my room now?" Glen said dully.

"Get him out of here," Stirewalt growled to an aide. "Get him out before he contaminates the place." He stuck a big finger in Glen's face and said, "I'll finish with you later, buster." Walking back across the gym, he frowned at the idle patients. "Okay, back to work. Come on, Billy, get on it. Mrs. Moore, let's go, work that shoulder." He clapped his hands together loudly. "Come on now."

"What the hell was that all about?" I said.

"You didn't see what he did?"

"No," I said, puzzled. "What?"

"He was faking. The dumb ass." Stirewalt chuckled, without a trace of anger. "He forgot to—"

"Shame on you, Mr. Stirewalt, shame on you."

We looked up from our conversation at Mrs. Blanche Overcash, an elderly lady, the victim of a stroke. She leaned heavily on her walker and looked sternly at Stirewalt. "You shouldn't use that kind of language around ladies and children. It's wrong. And that poor young man—you should be ashamed of yourself," she said.

"Yes, ma'am, I know but—"

"No buts about it," she continued. "It's wrong. You shouldn't do that."

"I'm sorry about that, Mrs. Overcash. I don't know what

81

got into me. I guess it's this vile Yankee temper of mine. I'll try to keep it under control from now on. You go on and apologize to the folks for me. Will you do that?"

"I'd be pleased to. But you simply must do something about that awful temper of yours."

"Yes. I will. I will."

We watched her make her way slowly out of hearing range as I whispered, "Shame on you."

Stirewalt shook his head slowly.

"You really ought to do something about that temper of yours."

He reached over and grabbed a tuft of hair on my calf and jerked it out.

"*Aughhhh*, son-of-a-*bitch*," I screamed.

"Shame on you." Stirewalt grinned.

"Okay, okay," I said. "How'd you know Glen was faking?"

"He forgot to stop chewing his gum. You didn't notice that?"

"No." I laughed.

"He's been faking all along. He should have been off that table long ago. You see, if he passes out, they take him back to his room and that's it for the day. So every day he comes in here for ten minutes, passes out, and bingo."

"Have you tried talking to him? I mean, really explaining it all to him?"

"I've tried everything; talking, crying, begging, threats—nothing. I'm working on fear right now. Maybe I can scare him into trying. If he thinks I'm gonna go beserk and get violent, then maybe . . ."

"What's wrong with that guy anyway? I mean, he doesn't talk to anybody and he keeps his head covered all the time. He has the sheet fixed so he can peek out and watch TV, but it's like he doesn't want anybody to see him or something."

"He's got some real problems. I mean, besides the obvious physical ones. He'd have problems even if he hadn't broken his neck. Have you met his father, J.B.?"

"No."

"Well, you're in for a treat. He's something else. Caused a hell of a mess around here," Stirewalt said, looking at the floor and shaking his head in disbelief. Looking over the thick frames of his glasses, he said. "He's crazy. Really. He's dangerous. He belongs to some crackpot religious outfit. Thinks Glen's being punished for some sin. That's part of Glen's problem; he doesn't want to go home. Try lifting that leg again."

I gripped the arm of the wheelchair with weak hands and strained against the weight of my leg.

"They're very poor," Stirewalt continued. "Tenant farmers, I believe. Glen knows he's not going to get very much return, but he's afraid he'll get enough to be released to his parents' care. He would prefer going to a nursing home. At least there he would have a TV and three good meals a day, and he would have some care. If he goes home he's just going to lie there in a shack. So what do you do?" Stirewalt shrugged. "Aren't you due in whirlpool?"

"Yes, in fifteen minutes."

"Well, come on back when you're finished and we'll work on your hands awhile."

I moaned. "My hands are fine, just weak. The more I use 'em the stronger they'll get."

"Can you touch your thumb and your little finger?" he asked solemnly.

I grimaced. "I hate that. I really do. It's frustrating and it takes so damn much effort, and when I do it I won't feel like I've accomplished anything."

"I know, but it's necessary, believe me," he said, slapping me on the knee. "I'll get an aide to run you over to hydrotherapy."

7

I SAT with my back to the wall, watching the patients around me, and worked the muscles of my arms and shoulders against the measured weight of the pulleys. I was trying to guess the causes for the variety of physical problems I saw before me. In the past month I had learned that stroke victims were affected on one side of the body only and walked with a distinctive shuffle, dragging one leg and supporting themselves awkwardly with one hand on a multi-tipped cane or walker, the other hand, suspended in a sling, dangling uselessly at their waist. Those whose heavily braced legs were swung in unison through supporting crutches were either polio victims or paraplegics whose condition resulted from a low spinal injury; it was hard for me to distinguish them. The sudden, violently jerking spasms caused by multiple sclerosis were easily recognizable, while the physical problems caused by brain surgery were so varied it would have been impossible for me to guess their cause were it not for the obvious scars left by the surgery. The game of trying to diagnose each patient never lost its fascination for me, and I was constantly asking Stirewalt questions to break the monotonous routine of repeated exercises.

84

I was watching one of the children stubbornly fighting to keep a therapist from putting a protective helmet on him when an aide came over and told me that Stirewalt would not be in; he had fallen off his bicycle and broken his leg.

I looked at her with astonishment. "He fell off his *bicycle?*"

"Yes," she snickered.

"What was he doing on a bicycle?"

"He rides it to work. Keeps his weight down," she explained.

"Well, how did he manage to—"

"Who knows." She shrugged. "It's just a hairline fracture. They didn't even admit him, just cast it and sent him home. He'll be in as soon as the cast hardens, probably tomorrow. He said for you to go through your usual routine, said you'd know what to do."

"I can just see him on a bicycle." I chuckled. "Like a trained bear. I'll bet he's got one of those skinny little English bikes, too."

"He does," she said with a conspiratorial grin. "I've seen him and that's exactly what he looks like—a trained bear." She giggled and went off across the gym.

Stirewalt had proved true to his word—he had worked me beyond anything I thought possible, but it had never been necessary for him to push. There had developed between us a friendly rivalry, a camaraderie that would not permit me to admit to exhaustion or give in to pain. If Stirewalt wanted to add two pounds of weight or pressure to a particular exercise, I insisted on four, and we argued incessantly over whether I could handle one weight or another or how long it would be until I could. I usually came out on top in these arguments, and Stirewalt was openly perplexed over my day-to-day progress, unaware that I had smuggled, one by one, a set of weights back to my room and spent a large part of each evening and night feverishly working up to the amount of weight that had been the subject of that day's disagreement. Except for an hour in hydrotherapy, I spent the entire day in the gym, although I was scheduled for only one hour of physical therapy each morning and each afternoon. I had refused to continue occupational therapy, feeling that the time could be better spent in the gym. "I'm not going to waste my time building some silly-ass birdhouse," I told Stirewalt and, to the administration's consternation, he had agreed and would advise me on various exercises between his regularly scheduled patients.

Almost one-fourth of the gym consisted of elevated mats raised to a height that allowed easy access from wheelchairs. I was lying on my back on one of the mats, patiently raking the heel of my left foot back and forth across a plywood board that had been sprinkled heavily with baby powder. The powder was supposed to reduce friction and lessen the wear on my heel. The range of my leg's lateral movement was clearly visible in the smooth graceful arc traced by my heel in the powder. I had been trying for an hour to extend this range, to lengthen the arc each time I moved my leg out and away from my body. As I shifted my body around to begin the same procedure on my right leg, I saw Stirewalt enter the gym. He walked in skillfully on new crutches and was immediately the center of attention. After being welcomed back and ribbed by his fellow workers and a few nearby patients, he propped his crutches against the wall and busied himself with a patient. He carefully avoided looking in my direction, and I continued my exercise, watching him out of the corner of my eye. It was almost an hour before he picked up his crutches and crossed the gym.

I looked up at him sorrowfully. "Ahhh, did it hurt its leg?"

"No," he said blankly, "why do you ask?"

I dropped my eyes to the cast on Stirewalt's left leg. "Well, I couldn't help noticing that you're either wearing a cast or one hell of a sweat sock."

"Oh, this," he said, looking down at the cast. "Funny you should notice."

"Yeah, well, I'm funny that way."

"This," he explained proudly, "is a cast."

"No! I'll be damned. So that's a cast? I thought you were beginning to petrify."

"No, no. It's a cast. You see, I've got a friend in med school," he said, "and he's learning to put on casts and I let him practice on me. He hasn't learned to take them off yet. He won't get to that course for six more weeks, but when he does"—he smiled triumphantly—"he's going to practice by taking this off."

"That's really big of you. Not just anybody would walk around in a cast for six weeks just so a friend could get in a little practice."

"I know," Stirewalt agreed, "I'm all heart."

"I wouldn't go that far," I said. "In fact, if you expect me to believe that story I'd have to say you're all ass."

"Now, is that any way to talk?" He pouted. "Is that nice?"

"As far as I can remember it was."

"As far as you can remember?"

"As far as I can remember her name was Linda."

"Whose name was Linda?"

"It was big and soft and beautiful."

"What was?"

"And it was nice then."

"What was nice? When? What the hell are you talking about?"

"Linda's ass. It was nice. What are you talking about?"

"I was talking about my leg."

"Ahhh, did it hurt its leg?"

Stirewalt winced. "Speaking of ass."

"Who's speaking of ass?"

"I am!" Stirewalt insisted. "Now get off yours and meet me at the parallel bars."

"We gonna *walk?*" I asked excitedly.

"That's all I've heard for the last week. Now if you've changed your mind, if you don't think you're ready—"

"I'm *ready*. I'm *ready*," I cried. "It's like I was telling Bo, you're all heart." I reached out my hand. He grasped it firmly and pulled, sliding me across the mat until my legs dropped over the edge and I came to a sitting position. I looked up at him expectantly. "Well, you going to help me with my shoes or not?"

"You'll have to put 'em on yourself."

"You know I can't do that," I told him. "I can't get down there with this brace on and if I could bend over I wouldn't be able to see my feet."

"Well, I can't get down there either with this cast on." A deep, low laugh rumbled through his massive chest. "The blind leading the blind. I'll get an aide."

At the parallel bars, he wrapped a wide canvas sash around my waist and tied it securely in back. He propped his crutches against the back of the wheelchair and moved to one side, slipped one hand under my arm, and took a firm grip on the back of the canvas sash. "Okay, let's see if you can stand up," he said, lifting the sash and my arm simultaneously.

"Wait a minute," I cried. "Hold on. Let me see if I can get up on my own."

"No way, hard nose. I think your legs will support you once you're up, but they're not strong enough to get you up there."

"They'll get me up," I assured him.

"They won't, I'm telling you."

"I say they will."

"And I'm telling you they won't."

"Stand back, give me room," I said, shaking his hand off my arm with a flourish. "A man's gotta have room to work."

"All right, all right," he said, shaking his head tiredly. "But you're going to bust your ass."

I reached for the parallel bars and pulled myself to the edge of my chair. I let go of the bars and took my right leg in my hands, just below the knee, and positioned it so that my foot was under me at an angle that would direct the pressure of my push to the ball of my foot, just behind the toes. Then I positioned my left leg and foot. Wiping the palms of my hands on my shorts, I inhaled deeply. Reaching again for the bars, I nervously fingered the polished wood, searching with my palms and fingers for a workable grip. Tightening my fingers, I locked my hands firmly to the bars and pulled. The new muscles of my arms and shoulders tensed, strained, and stood out clearly defined and taxed as I slid forward out of the chair and hung, suspended, motionless on the balls of my feet. The stringy muscles of my legs strained and throbbed and trembled under my weight. Time stopped. I was frozen there. I pulled with my arms and tried with all of my strength to force my legs to straighten. The untested muscles of my legs could not lift me and would not long support me. I stubbornly refused to sink. Sweat popped out across my face, down my rapidly tiring arms, and on my trembling, laboring legs. I drove my feet into the floor with all the force I could muster. My legs began to straighten, slowly. My body began a creeping upward journey from its crouched position. Both legs began to shake. I tried to ease back on my feet, to get off my toes, to get my feet flat on the floor. The calf of my left leg began shaking violently, harder and faster, until it was sliding my foot forward in short jerky spurts. I tried to stop it by shifting my weight to my right leg. My right leg began shaking in protest to the added strain. I felt myself tilt to the right and could feel myself going down, heading for the bar and the floor. I let go with my hands and kicked out hard with my right foot, harder than I thought possible, propelling myself backward into the wheelchair. I sat there soaked with sweat, gasping for breath.

"I told you," Stirewalt said with a superior smirk.

"I'm not through," I puffed.

"You're wasting your time," he insisted, "and you're going to overtax your legs."

"No, I'm not," I explained. "I figured out what I did wrong. I tried to come up slow and steady, on my toes. I've got to come up hard and fast and flat-footed."

"Look," he pleaded, "I know how much weight we've been working with on your leg exercises and I know approximately how heavy you are—there ain't no way."

"If I come up too fast I might get overbalanced and pitch forward on my face. Get a good grip on that belt," I told him. "If I come up too fast and get overbalanced you're going to have to hold me back."

Stirewalt stared at me with a big, fascinated grin. "I don't believe it. You're crazy, Tom. A minute ago your legs wouldn't even hold you up and now you're worried about coming up so fast I'll have to hold you back."

I ignored him and pulled myself to the edge of the chair. I took several deep breaths, slapped my hands down loudly on the bars, locked my fingers into the hard, smooth wood, and pulled myself forward out of the chair. In that fraction of a second, as the chair gave up my weight and just before my legs accepted it, I lunged forward by pulling hard on the bars with the stringent muscles of my arms and shoulders. At the same time, I drove my feet solidly into the floor and pushed determinedly, the muscles of my legs hardening, drawing into tight quivering knots as I began a torpid ascent. I began to rise faster, my legs straightening under me. I was halfway there and I was going to make it. Sudden powerful shimmers came up through my body, hammering my chin against the brace in a succession of rapid jolts. My legs were shaking violently. I had pitched forward onto my toes. I pressed my feet flat onto the floor, rocked back on my heels, and pushed myself upward, pulling with my arms. My legs straightened and stiffened. I felt my knees lock as I pitched forward, carried by my momentum. I slid my right hand forward on the bar to brace myself just as Stirewalt pulled back firmly on the sash and placed a huge steadying hand on my shoulder.

I was up. I was standing with my legs spread securely under me, my hands braced against the bars. It was a wondrous sensation. It was the most glorious feeling I had ever known. But it was more than just a feeling. It was freedom. The rigid bars of my imprisoning body were crumbling. I was free. Free of wrinkled beds and cold mats and confining wheelchairs. Free of irascible nurses and obstinate orderlies and stifling regimen. Free of fear. Free of the nagging, persistent, nightmarish fear that my faith in myself would prove false. I looked out across the gym and the world. I savored the warm, glowing tingle of new life coursing through me, the intoxicating headiness of the moment. Then I put it behind me. Stirewalt was at my side, his huge fist tenaciously gnarled in the canvas sash. I smiled triumphantly at him. "And they said it couldn't be done."

"I've got to hand it to you," he said with a broad grin, "I didn't think you could do it. And you're taller than I thought," he said, looking at me appraisingly. "How tall are you?"

"A little under six feet," I replied, "but I feel like a giant. I feel like I'm standing on the edge of a cliff and the floor is a thousand feet away. Man, it seems like that floor is a *long* way off."

Stirewalt chuckled. "Well, stand up straight," he demanded.

"I am straight."

"You're leaning to the right."

"I'm leaning to the right?"

"You're leaning to the right," he said flatly. "Straighten up. Come on. A little more to the left. A little more. *There.* Hold it. Now you're straight."

"I'm leaning to the left," I argued.

"You're straight!"

"I'm leaning to the left, I tell you."

"You're crazy. You're straight as an arrow."

"My right hand's the only thing keeping me up," I told him. "If I let go with my right hand I'll fall over the left bar."

Stirewalt muttered to himself as he swung down under the bar and came up in front of me. He eyed me carefully, frowning intently. "Jesus H. Christ, it's that damn brace again. It's got your head cocked to the left. It's not noticeable when you're sitting or lying down because you compensate by leaning to the right. I've had it with that piece of junk. Here, sit back down," he said, holding me under each arm and easing me back into the chair. I'll be back in a minute. I'm going to call Dr. Walters right now and get rid of that thing." He picked up his crutches and swung out of the gym.

When he came back he was carrying a shiny white plastic collar. He leaned his crutches against the parallel bars and began unbuckling the leather straps on my shoulders. "Dr. Walters said it wasn't necessary to wear this any longer. I thought you'd had the damn thing on long enough, and it's nothing but a goddamn nuisance. This collar should do the job just fine," he said as he unsnapped the metal latch at my left cheek and slid the heavy brace off my shoulders. Although I did not have to wear the brace in bed, I had never been up without it. This was the first time my neck had had to support the weight of my head unaided. I sat motionless, afraid that a move, however slight, would shift the weight of my head to an angle that my neck could not support. I felt naked, dangerously vulnerable and exposed. I had hated that heavy, awkward brace and had looked forward to being rid of it, but now I missed the security it had provided. Stirewalt snapped the light, sturdy collar around my neck.

"There, how does that feel?" he asked.

"Are you sure this thing gives me enough support?"

"It doesn't give you any support. You don't need support. You need protection from sudden movement. You need something to keep you from moving your neck too fast or too far, and this is just the ticket." He reached down, taking me by one arm and the back of the sash, and lifted me effortlessly to my feet. "Now, let's see you walk."

I expected my legs automatically to carry me smoothly down the long narrow alley formed by the bars, and when nothing happened, I was surprised and a little confused. I tried to remember exactly how to go about walking. It was something I had never consciously thought of before. Walking had been second nature, never requiring any thought. It was not going to be so simple now. I was going to have to consciously work individual muscles and groups of muscles in synchronization. I decided to use the muscles of my thigh to lift my leg and then whatever muscles were necessary to extend my leg from the knee. I gripped the bar and brought my right leg forward and up and then pushed my foot forward, straightening the leg. My toe caught the floor and dragged. I had done something wrong. I was sure I had raised my leg high enough to clear my foot. Of course, how stupid could I be. My foot. I had forgotten about my foot. I had left it dangling at the end of my leg. Of course it dragged. I had to get my toes up so the foot would clear the floor and my heel would touch down first as I stepped forward. I flexed the muscles of my left thigh, bringing my knee up at the same time I brought up the toes of my left foot. My weight shifted to my right leg as I extended my left foot and stepped forward. My right hip swung out to the right and I was overbalanced, crashing into the bar. I regained my balance and tried again with my right leg, being careful to remember to raise my foot. Again as I stepped forward, my weight shifted and I was overbalanced to the left, stopping only when my hip hit the bar.

I decided to try it faster, to take two quick steps and get through the hip movement before I lost my balance. I brought my right leg up and forward as fast as I could and felt my toe scrape but I ignored it, feeling my left hip giving to the left. I planted my right foot and leaned into it as I brought my left leg forward. My right hip swayed and lightly touched the bar.

"Whoa, hold on," Stirewalt cried. "You're swinging your hips like a drunk whore. Look, when you step forward you commit all your weight to one leg, you come forward *on* that leg. When you do, it's natural for the hip to swing out a little, but *just* a little," he explained. "You're going to have to control how much. You're letting your weight force your hip out from under you. Let your hip go just a little, then check it. Stop it before it's gone too far."

I looked at him as if he had just asked me to fly. "How can I do all that in the middle of a single step?"

"All what? Just control your hip. Quit worrying about falling. I've got you."

"Quit worrying about falling? Who's worried about falling? I haven't had time to think about that yet. I'm trying to tell everything what to do, and get it all in order, and make it all come out at the same time. I've got a thigh and a knee and a calf and a foot that won't do a damn thing unless I tell a specific muscle what to do. I'm trying to get one muscle to tense and another to relax at the same time, and now you want me to check my hips." I laughed and shook my head. "Would you like for me to sing your favorite song as I walk along?"

"No." He chuckled. "I don't think I could stand it. You won't have to think about every little move once you get a pattern going. So for now, do what you can about those hips or you won't ever get to a pattern."

I leaned forward into another step and dragged my toe, ignored it, and tried hard to stop my hip as it began to swing out from under me. I stopped it before it reached the bar. By the time I made my third trip down the parallel bars I was clearing my feet with a steady regularity and keeping my hips within a workable range, although they still swung in an exaggerated fashion.

"Let's make another trip and then knock off for a while," Stirewalt suggested.

"Sounds good to me," I panted.

"You've got damn good foot placement, heel and toe, heel and toe, it's looking good. I'd say you'll be on crutches in two weeks or so."

I looked at him with a slow smile. "I'd say a week at the most."

8

THE sweat running profusely off my face matted my hair, plastering it to my forehead in tight ringlets. It ran in a steady stream down my temples and glistened on the darkly throbbing vein ridging down my forehead. I could not straighten my leg. I was lying on my back with my right leg drawn up so that my foot was flat against the mat. I thought about forcing my leg down with one of the crutches at my side, but decided against it. I had been trying for forty-five minutes to straighten that leg and, by God, I was going to do it. It had been a week since I had first walked in the parallel bars, and today I had used crutches for the first time. It had exhausted me and I had stopped here to rest, intending to stay for only a few minutes, but my leg, drawn up absently for comfort as I watched the activities of the gym, stubbornly refused to be moved.

The effort was draining the last of my energy, and my frustration flared into searing anger. "You'll stay in here till you rot! It's almost dinnertime, but I'll keep you in here till you starve. You're going to move and you're going to move on your own. I'm not going to do it for you, not with my hands and not with crutches or anything else. Now move!" I hissed in a voice seething with frustration. I mounted a massive effort, straining every muscle in my body. My foot dug deep into the mat as the tightened muscles of my stomach pulled me almost to a sitting position. I hung there, my entire body trembling from the heart-cracking effort. My leg refused to move and I glared at it with a cold, naked hatred for a moment before I relaxed and fell back on the mat, panting. "You stubborn, hard-headed, half-assed, rat bastard son-of-a-bitch," I gasped.

"Who you talking to?" asked Stirewalt, looking around the gym. I had not seen him come over to the mats.

"Nobody," I said self-consciously.

He looked at me suspiciously, then slowly moved his eyes to my leg. "You were talking to your leg, weren't you?"

"No."

"Yes you were." He smiled. "You were talking to your leg. I'll be damned."

"At least I don't go around falling off bicycles and breaking mine."

"You're probably afraid it will stop talking to you if you do."

"Well, the damn thing won't work. I've been stuck here for a goddamn hour."

"What's wrong with it?"

"I don't know what's wrong with it," I told him. "I can't straighten it out."

"Well, let's have a look," he said, moving down the mat for a closer look. "Try it now."

I took a deep breath and labored to straighten my leg. My foot pressed hard against the mat, raising my hip several inches. I arched my back and writhed my body, trying to break my foot loose from the mat. My hip began to quiver as the fatigued muscles dropped me back to the mat.

"Well, no wonder," he said. "You're not *trying* to straighten your leg."

"Not trying?" I gasped. "Not trying? No! I've been lying here for an hour enjoying myself. What do you mean—not trying?"

"I mean you're not trying to straighten your leg. You're trying hard enough, but you're trying to push your foot *through* the mat, not *down* it. Did you notice how your hip came up?"

"Yeah."

"Well, that's because you're pushing your foot straight down into the mat. You're using your thigh and hip muscles and you're driving all the force straight into the mat," Stirewalt explained. "You've got to do just the opposite. Use your hip to lift your leg, get the pressure off your foot and your foot off the mat. Then use your thigh to bring your foot forward just like you were trying to kick something. Try it."

I eyed him tiredly for a moment, then braced for the effort. I was surprised to find little effort required. My leg straightened out smooth and easy. "Well, I'll be damned."

"You should be, but we don't have time. Dr. Walters wants to see you in the conference room."

"Is anything wrong?"

"No, I don't think so. He just wants to see you," he said. "Do you want to try to walk down there or ride?"

"I'll walk," I said, sitting on the edge of the mat struggling to tie my shoe. I took Stirewalt's arm and pulled myself to my feet. Stirewalt slipped a crutch under each of my arms and moved behind me, hooking two fingers through my belt and grabbing the handle of a wheelchair with his free hand. I started across the gym, taking short, choppy steps. I locked my knees on each step and my hips were still unreliably loose. Stirewalt followed close behind, still holding my belt and towing the wheelchair.

When we reached the conference room at the end of a long corridor, my legs were wobbly and my breath was coming in short puffs. Stirewalt swung the chair around and steadied me as I collapsed into it. He held the crutches in one hand and pushed the door open with the other.

"I'll keep the crutches," I puffed.

"Oh, no, I'll keep 'em in the gym. I don't want you trying to walk unless I'm with you." He smiled knowingly. "I wouldn't want you practicing in your room."

98

I rolled the wheelchair into the room and saw Dr. Walters standing in the far corner holding an X-ray up to the light. He was a tall, dignified man whom I would have guessed to be in his late forties or early fifties. His silver-gray hair made him appear older and gave him an air of authority. His clothes were always impeccably tailored and perfectly color-coordinated. I wondered how he could put in a full day and still look as though he had just finished dressing. His eyes were soft and compassionate, lacking the piercing intellect of Dr. McKinnon's. His manner was warm and friendly, and I had absolute confidence in him.

"I was just looking at some of your X-rays," he said, turning and crossing the room.

"Is anything wrong?" I asked nervously.

"No, no, I don't think so," he said. "How are you getting along?"

"Fine. It's coming along pretty good," I told him. I was still ill at ease. Dr. Walters always came by my room. There had to be a reason for being in the conference room.

"I hear you're on crutches now."

"Yes. It's slow but it's coming."

"You'll be out of here before you know it if you keep that up." He chuckled.

"Yes, I guess so. I hope so," I replied. I wished he would get to the point.

Dr. Walters snapped off the collar and rotated my head gently in a circle, searching with his hands. He pressed lightly on the back of my neck and tilted my head, first forward then backward. "How's the sensation?"

"Good. Real good. Normal, I guess."

"No change? You haven't noticed any change lately, have you?"

"No."

"How about the neck? Much pain?"

"No more than usual. Maybe a little less, or maybe I'm just getting used to it."

"Any spasms?"

"No."

"You're not on any medication now, are you?" he said, snapping the collar back in place.

"No, nothing. Well, vitamins."

He was silent as he checked my reflexes; then he pulled up a chair and sat down facing me. He looked at me seriously for a long moment, then said, "I've been in touch with Dr. McKinnon about your last set of X-rays, and he doesn't feel that your neck is as stable as it could be. As a precaution, he's suggesting an anterior fusion."

"Anterior fusion?" I frowned. "That means an operation. From the front?"

"It's a new procedure they've come up with in neurology. It's fusing the front of the vertebrae, and in order to do this it's necessary to go in through the throat. Because of the high-risk factor, there is some strong disagreement between those of us in orthopedic medicine and the neurosurgeons as to the relative merits of this particular piece of surgery."

"What kind of risk does it involve?"

"You're taking a risk any time you go into surgery, and doubly so when you're dealing with the spinal cord. There is always the possibility that you could suffer the loss of some function, either partially or completely, and I believe that this possibility is too great with this particular procedure."

"Is there another procedure that you recommend? I mean, if I need this fusion, what choice do I have?"

"You've asked me two questions. First, no, there isn't another procedure. The entire field of neurosurgery is relatively new. They're feeling their way along and making fantastic progress. Just a few years ago if you broke your neck you died; there just wasn't any surgery available. So, quite a lot of what they're doing is new and there just aren't that many alternatives.

"Now as to your other question, whether or not you need it. Dr. McKinnon and I are agreed that your neck is stable,

100

but he wants the added precaution of an anterior fusion. I don't feel that it's necessary, not at this time anyway. If it becomes necessary later, and I don't think it will, it can be done then. I've consulted three of my colleagues, two here and one in Chicago, and they're of the opinion that there is nothing in your X-rays that would warrant the risk of surgery. These are top men, but you should feel free to consult anyone you like, get several more opinions if you like, talk it over with your folks."

"No, I don't think that'll be necessary. You say it can be done later if it has to be?"

"Yes, if there is some indication that the posterior fusion Dr. McKinnon did is no longer providing the desired stability, then we can take the necessary steps to achieve that stability."

"It doesn't make sense to risk losing the use of an arm or leg just to prevent something that *might* happen, especially not if it can be corrected when and if it ever happens," I said.

"That's the way we feel about it, but of course Dr. McKinnon sees it differently."

I shook my head. "No, I don't want to take that risk, not now."

That night after dinner I lay in bed toying with the dumbbells and brooding. It wasn't like Dr. McKinnon to take any chances, to risk anything. He just would not do it. There must really be a need for that operation if he suggested it. But if that was true, why didn't the other doctors see it? And if it could wait until the need was evident to all, why was McKinnon in such a hurry? Maybe it boiled down to the procedure itself. They agreed my neck was stable, and McKinnon just wanted to hedge his bet. As a neurosurgeon, he used the procedure and did not consider it to be of a high-risk factor, while Walters did not use it and thought the risk too high. That had to be it. McKinnon wanted to give me the added protection of an anterior fusion and felt he could do it without risking the loss of anything. But, as Walters said, any surgery was dangerous.

I would not take the chance of being paralyzed again. McKinnon's intentions were good, but Walters was right. Why take the chance if you don't have to?

I heard a commotion in the hall and recognized Rick's laugh and the deep rumbling guffaw of Herb Brockman. I was glad they had come. I had decided to go with Dr. Walters' opinion on the fusion, and now I would like to forget it. It would be good to see Herb again. I had not seen him since we had all gotten drunk together at the New Year's Eve party. Rick and I had met Herb for the first time when we went out for peewee football, and we had played ball together from that time all the way through high school. Over the years we had come to depend on Herb's steady blocking and thought nothing of lowering our heads and charging blindly into an opponent's line, knowing that somehow he would blast a hole for us.

"Hey, you ol' cock biter. How's it going?" Herb asked as he and Rick strolled into the room.

"Not bad. Not bad at all," I answered, looking up at them. Herb was as big as Stirewalt. He had a full cupid's face and a broad, flat nose that had been broken more times than any of us could remember. His thick, tawny hair was an unkempt mass of curls.

"We can't stay but a minute. Rick says he knows a couple skirts that we can pick up. Probably a couple dogs," Herb said as he lapped a big hand over the back of a chair, spun it around, and straddled it. Rick hopped up on the foot of the bed and squirmed around, hunting a comfortable position.

"Who cares." I chuckled. "It's been so long I wouldn't care if she barked or not."

"If we find an extra one we'll bring her by for you," said Rick. "Think you can remember what to do?"

I laughed. "That's funny. That's funnier than you think. If it's anything like walking was for the first time, I'll never keep it all straight in my mind."

"You been in here too long," Herb said. "It ain't like walking. It ain't like walking at all."

102

I didn't hear him. I was wondering which muscles I would have to use and in what sequence. I found the prospect intriguing and wondered if I would manage it, and if I was able to get everything working in the right direction, at the right time, and in proper sequence, whether I would be too busy to enjoy it. But then, by the time I had the opportunity to find out it would probably no longer be necessary consciously to direct individual muscles; it was getting to be less so every day.

"Well, we better score tonight," Herb said, looking at Rick. "I go back to school tomorrow and it'll be assholes and jock straps for the next three weeks."

"Football practice starting already?"

"Yeah." Herb grinned. "But what's this ol' slick tells me about you getting busted at the beach over Mother's Day weekend?"

"That's right," I said. "Did he tell you why?"

"It wasn't *my* fault," Rick insisted.

"The hell you yell. You're the one who hit that paratrooper."

"Well, I couldn't help it."

"You hit a *paratrooper?*" Herb asked, looking at Rick with mounting respect.

Rick shrugged helplessly. "Look, it was spring and we went down to the beach to watch the girls and hoping to get lucky," he explained. "The place was crawling with paratroopers. The Eighty-second Airborne was in town for something, and you couldn't move without bumping into one of those bastards. As soon as we got into that joint across from the pavilion, Tom spotted a blonde and cut a trail for her table, so I stepped up to the bar and started scouting the territory. Well, this big bruiser muscled in beside me and kinda bumped me, but I didn't say anything. Then he looked at my legs and said, 'You got likely legs.' I figured he was queer so I ignored him. Then he grinned real big and said, 'Likely to break off and stick up your ass.' I didn't know what to do, I mean, I didn't want any part of a paratrooper and besides he was a big son-of-a-bitch. So while I'm thinking it over, trying to figure out what

103

to do, he plops that goddamn big boot down on my bare foot and keeps right on grinning at me. So I hauled off and flattened his ass." Rick smiled proudly.

"And then what did you do?" Herb asked.

"He ran like hell," I said.

"You fucking A I ran. I was gonna stay and fight but that place exploded. It went crazy. People started throwing chairs and bottles, women were screaming, and those motherfucking paratroopers were jumping up on the tables and yelling. Damn right, I ran."

"I looked up about the time Rick cold-cocked that fucker," I said. "When I saw him start for the door—"

"You ran," Rick put in. "You turned around and ran right into a cop."

"Okay, so I ran. All I wanted to do in the first place was get out of there, but where do I end up? In the local lockup."

"How long were you locked up?" Herb laughed.

"Not long. They weren't interested in me. They wanted those paratroopers. They'd been raising hell all over town."

"What happened to you?" Herb asked Rick.

"I'll tell you what happened to him," I said. "When I got back to the motel about four o'clock that morning, that asshole there had me locked out and wouldn't let me in. He was shacked up in there with *my* blonde."

"Man does not live by bread alone," declared Rick.

"How'd you end up with her?" Herb asked.

"I was just sitting under that table watching all the action, and she came crawling under there."

"You didn't get hit at all?"

"Nope. Nobody laid a glove on me."

"If I could have gotten into that room I'd have laid one on you," I told him.

"I know, that's why you didn't get in." Rick smiled.

"You know what that son-of-a-bitch did?" I asked Herb. "He called the cops on me. On *me!*"

"Well, you set up such a howl out there you were gonna wake up the manager and get us all thrown out." Rick turned to Herb. "He was out there beating on the door, and cussing, and ranting and raving, and threatening to kill me. The girl got scared and said she was leaving. I had to do something."

"You didn't have to call the law," I said.

"I *told* you I called 'em. I told them there was a drunk out there creating a disturbance and to send a car over, then I told you to beat it out of there, the cops were coming."

"Did they come?" Herb asked.

"Damn right they came. I had to run like hell. The room was registered in his name and I knew that bastard would say he didn't know me from Adam." I looked at Rick. "That's one I owe you."

Rick winced.

We swapped more stories for a while, and then it was time for them to leave.

"Let's go," Rick said to Herb as he slid off the bed. "Let's go before he remembers something else. We're already late."

Herb stood up and turned the chair around. "Oh, did you ever figure out what the golden horse meant?"

"What golden horse?" I asked.

"The one in the vision?"

"What vision?"

"Aw, come on," he said. "I know all about it."

Behind him Rick held his hands out, palms up, and shrugged helplessly.

"Said you had it all figured out except the golden horse," Herb explained.

"Oh," I said, "you mean when my life flashed in front of me. No, I haven't figured it out yet."

"Well, let me know if you ever do. And try to come up for one of the games. Let me know which one, and I'll send you some tickets. If I don't see you then, I'll be home Christmas and we'll tie one on."

"Sounds good to me."

"I'll see you later," Rick called over his shoulder as they went out the door.

A golden horse! I wondered what kind of tale Rick had come up with.

9

I PLACED the cigarette between Bo's lips and leaned back in the chair. The lunch hour was almost over, and the gym would be open in a few minutes. I thought it was foolish to lock the gym during the lunch period. It didn't take a full hour to eat a hospital meal and I needed that time to work on my balance and coordination. The two canes I was using interfered with my rhythm and made it difficult to establish a steady gait. A little extra time in the gym was all that was needed to correct that.

"Does your neck hurt much?" asked Bo, the cigarette wagging up and down as he spoke.

I toyed with a loose string at the hem of my shorts. "Yeah, especially after I've been up awhile," I answered without looking up. Bo's eyes were disconcerting. Those opaque, lifeless eyes held unspoken accusations that filled me with guilt. I knew Bo hated me for recovering, and several times I had almost apologized, but each time anger prevented it. Dammit, I wasn't responsible for Bo's condition. My own injury was the result of an accident I had not caused or had any control over, but Bo's resulted from his own stupid actions. A child would have known better than to dive into water where the depth was unknown. That was goddamn stupid.

"You know the worst thing about being paralyzed?" Bo asked, not giving me a chance to answer. "It's feeling the same things, wanting the same things. You'd think that would change, but it doesn't. Somebody asked me once what it was like being paralyzed and I told him to imagine waking up one morning to find that his head had been severed from his body and placed on a shelf where it could watch life going on around it. He wasn't going to die and nothing in his life had changed, except that now he was just a head sitting on a shelf. I can never get it across to anyone that that head still has the same sex drive it always had even though there's no body to perform the act, that it still has the same ego and the same needs. I don't think anybody can ever really understand, do you?"

"No, I don't think so," I said, holding an ashtray beneath Bo's cigarette and knocking the ash into it.

"My wife used to sit on the side of the bed when she came to see me, and I wanted her as much as I ever had. She'd look so fresh and clean in a summer dress and I could smell her perfume, and without thinking about it I'd start to reach for her, and then it would hit me. For a moment I'd forgotten I was paralyzed, and realizing it again was like realizing it for the first time."

Settling back in the chair, I hoped Bo wasn't going to start talking about his wife. It would only depress us both, as it always did. Bo's wife seldom came to visit him, and Bo said he knew she had a lover and he didn't really blame her, but he did wish she'd bring his daughter by more often.

"What'd you think when you first woke up and realized you were paralyzed?" Bo asked.

"I don't know what I thought. I was so damn scared and I hurt so bad I just started looking around for the ol' panic button."

"Yeah, me too. I didn't think it was possible to hurt that bad and still live. Then when the panic hit me, my mind went wild. It was like my brain was jumping up and down and running around inside my head screaming to get out, and all I could do was hang on and wait for everything to calm down. But the pain was the worst part. If they hadn't kept me knocked out with those pain shots I'd be a raving lunatic today. Remember how bad it got when you had to wait an hour or more for the next shot?"

"I didn't take any shots. I found out early in the game that they made me sick. And I'll tell you something—I can't take being sick. If I get sick, I'll die on you. I can take pain a lot better than I can take being sick."

"It must not have been as bad for you as it was for me, or you'd have been begging for those shots."

"Maybe," I said, taking the cigarette from Bo's mouth and snuffing it out. "But it was bad enough that I knew I couldn't handle the pain and being sick both. Not and come out alive, I couldn't."

"I wanted to die. I just wanted out, and death was the quickest door. I *tried* to die."

"Not me. I wanted out, but I didn't want to die."

"You never wanted to die? Not once?"

"No."

"Then you couldn't have hurt the way I did. That kind of pain would make anybody want to die," Bo said bitterly.

"Yeah, I guess it would."

"Maybe you're just afraid to die. That's the difference, isn't it? You're afraid to die."

"No. I'm not afraid of death. I want to live. There are things I want bad enough to live for, that's all."

"What? What could be that important?"

"It's not important—not to anybody but me. There's just something I'd like to know before I die."

Bo grew thoughtful and watched me out of the corner of

109

his eye. "You can't tell me you didn't think about suicide when they told you you were going to be paralyzed for the rest of your life."

"No, I can't. I *did* think about it—once. Right after I moved my hand for the first time I began to think that was all the return I was going to get. So I started working like hell on that hand just in case."

"Well, we're not so different after all," Bo said tartly. "That's what I did when I first got some return in my shoulder. I figured if I could get the use of one hand, just one hand, then . . . but I never got that hand."

"I only thought about it that one time," I explained. "Then I decided that if I was going to beat it, I had to keep on believing it. I couldn't have any alternative goals. So I forgot about it."

"And what if you hadn't gotten any more return? You wouldn't have been able to forget about it so easily, would you?"

"I don't know." I shrugged.

"The hell you don't. You know damn well you'd still be lying there trying to figure a way out."

"I guess you're right," I conceded.

"You know I'm right," he insisted. "And if you'd never gotten that one hand? What then? How do you think you'd have done it?"

I looked at him with growing doubt and trepidation. "I don't know. I haven't thought about it."

"How much thought does it take? There's only one way, and you know it."

With sudden understanding, I looked up into eyes that overwhelmed me, that were filmed and clouded and pleading.

"Help me, Tom," he said in a frail, childlike voice.

"Bo, for God's sake."

"No, listen. All you have to do is tilt that bottle," he said, nodding toward a bottle of IV fluid hanging above him. "Just tilt it enough to allow air to get into the tube. That's all. Just tilt the bottle."

110

"I can't, Bo. I'm sorry. I just can't."

"Tom, you know what it's like being locked up in your own body. That's the worst kind of prison. You'd want me to do it for you."

I exhaled slowly and was silent for a moment, remembering. "Yes, I'd want you to do it for me."

"You know the life expectancy of a quad. Seven years. That means I've got five more years. Five years of nothing. Five years of waiting. Waiting for a blood clot to come floating up out of a leg and hit something vital, or for a kidney to fail, or for pneumonia. Five years, Tom. *Five years!* Please, for God's sake, get me off this shelf."

I stared at the floor, not wanting to look into those eyes. "I can't. I know I'd want you to do it for me. I'd beg you to do it, but I can't."

"Nobody'll know. It'll be instantaneous. They'll think it was a blood clot and even if they don't, they'll figure some nurse made a mistake."

I continued to stare at the floor and slowly shook my head.

"What the hell are you afraid of?" he cried. "Not them! Not being caught. It's something else." He bit his trembling lip and carefully studied me. I could feel his eyes. "I've heard you pray. Is that it? Is that what you're afraid of?"

I looked up helplessly.

"You can still believe that? After what you've been through? After what you've seen?" he moaned in a voice filled with misery and disdain. "Are you blind? Look around you. Take a good hard look at the rotting flesh and the twisted bodies of the human wreckage lying around here, and then tell me what you believe."

"I have looked, and I can't explain it or justify it or make any sense out of it. But Bo, locked up inside of yourself haven't you realized that we're more than flesh and bone, that there is something in us that's a part of something bigger?"

"No! I'll tell you what I've realized; there's pain and there's loneliness and there's fear, but there ain't no God. It's a fairy tale! A lie! And you're a fool to believe that garbage. A fool afraid of Santa Claus."

"No, not Santa Claus and not the all-forgiving, benevolent Old Man of the church, Bo. I don't know much about God, but I do know that we're a part of something, we belong to something, and it's big. It's the biggest, most awesome force in the universe. And you're right, I am afraid of it. I'd be a fool *not* to be," I said, standing up slowly and reaching for the canes propped against the bedside cabinet.

"But not so afraid that you wouldn't have ended your own miserable life." He sneered.

"That was different."

"Different because it was you and not me."

"No, different because of my reason for dying. I wasn't going to end my life to escape. I wasn't going to do it for myself. It was for my family. I wasn't going to let their lives be ruined by a lifetime of hospital bills. I wasn't going to watch them do without all they had worked for and dreamed of and wanted. It was for them. And I think God or anybody else could forgive that."

"What I'm asking you to do is the same thing. It's not for you. It's for me. You'd be doing it for someone else."

"It's not the same thing, Bo. You're not giving me anything."

"Giving you anything?" he cried in a thick, infuriated voice. "What the hell can I give you? What do you want from me?"

"A reason! A reason I can live with or, more important, a reason I can die with," I explained. "If I loved you enough, I could do it. I could live with that. If I loved you enough, I could forgive myself, but I don't and I'm sorry." I turned awkwardly and walked slowly toward the door.

"You son-of-a-bitch! You chickenshit son-of-a-bitch!" he screamed in a voice quavering with exasperation. "You remember me, hear? Think of me every time you take a step. Every time you move from one place to another, remember me and remember what it's like, you bastard. You goddamn bastard!"

I turned the corner and started down the long empty hall. I tried to ignore Bo's frustrated, angry screams but I couldn't. I snagged a toe and to keep from falling I jammed my shoulder into the wall and hung there with my eyes closed. I would have wanted Bo to do it for me. Maybe that was reason enough, I thought. Maybe I should have done it.

"Are you all right?" a nurse asked.

I glanced up and, without answering, pushed myself upright and moved off down the hall.

When I entered the gym I was relieved to find no one using the bicycle. It was the most active exercise available and I needed activity now. I didn't want to think. I had often used the bicycle to blindly grind out anger, driving my legs until exhaustion washed away frustration.

I adjusted the tension on the bike and began working my legs while absently watching the gym fill slowly with patients and tried not to think of Bo. Damn him. Sure I would have wanted him to do it for me, but I would never have asked. I would have figured some way to do it, and that's what Bo would have to do. Damn him.

Stirewalt, leaning heavily on a cane, came in limping. His cast had been removed the previous day to the delight of his patients, who readily offered suggestions as to how he could improve his walking pattern. When one of the paraplegics expressed exaggerated sympathy for Stirewalt's condition, I felt my mood begin to lighten. Then I remembered Bo's eyes and the murky clouds floating deep beneath their surface. I felt a shiver pass through me as I furiously drove my legs and swore it would never happen to me. Nothing would ever beat me that completely. Nothing would ever choke the life out of me like that.

I continued pedaling as hard and as fast as I could, ticking off mile after creeping mile on the odometer, until my legs were jabbing at the pedals rather than pushing them around with a steady, controlled force. Breathing deeply, I wiped the

113

sweat off my face and slid off the bike. Steadying myself with the canes, I stood for a moment enjoying the warm, glowing tingle in my legs before moving to the corner of the gym.

I had never known the intended purpose for the series of wooden bars that ran ladderlike up the wall in this neglected corner. They were about four feet long and spaced six inches apart, covering the wall all the way to the ceiling.

Holding to one of the bars for balance, I began doing knee bends, pausing in the middle of each one, forcing my legs to support my motionless weight for a few seconds before continuing. I was pleased with my progress, especially my legs. They were growing stronger daily and filling out rapidly. When the muscles were swollen and puffed by exercise, my legs were almost the size they had been before the accident.

"Move over and I'll join you," said Stirewalt. "I've got to work the kinks out of this leg sometime."

I moved over without saying anything and Stirewalt stepped up to the bars. Continuing the exercise, I thought the barely audible sounds were coming from a nearby patient, but there were no patients in this area of the gym. Listening more intently, I realized the anguished moans were coming from beside me. Comprehension dawned slowly as I looked with stunned disbelief at Stirewalt, who was grimacing fiercely although he had gotten only a quarter of the way into a knee bend.

"Well, I'll be damned," I said.

"What?" he said self-consciously.

"You pussy! You big *pussy!*"

"What the hell are you talking about?"

"You! You're what I'm talking about, pussy. Moaning and groaning and making faces like some little girl. You aren't wearing lace panties are you, chubby cheeks?"

"Listen, acid mouth, trying to bend this knee for the first time in six weeks ain't no fun. It happens to be painful as hell, and you can't rush it."

114

"Tell me about it. How about all those times you tried to tear my leg off? You don't think that was painful?"

"That was different. I'm not in any hurry and you said you were, and besides, you've got a high pain threshold. You're not normal."

"Bullshit! I hurt just like you. You're the one who's odd. Just put your weight on that leg. Let your weight force it down."

"Are you crazy?" he said with a look of scorn. "I'm not going to risk tearing some cartilage."

"Don't give me that." I laughed. "You can't tear cartilage by bending your knee in the direction it's suppose to bend. That's the worst excuse I've ever heard. Put your weight on it. Go on."

With a sneer, he repositioned himself at the bars and began to shift his weight gently to his still leg. It began to bend slowly under the added weight. With a sudden moan he grimaced and jerked himself to a standing position. He gave me a menacing look to show that the blame rested with me.

"Don't ease up," I said, smothering a laugh. "If you—"

"Would you just go on and let me handle this."

"Well, you're not going to accomplish very much easing off every time it hurts."

"It's a reflex action," he snapped. "It's natural! It's normal! But you wouldn't know about that, would you?"

"What are you yelling at me for?"

"I'm not yelling at you," he yelled.

"Look," I said, moving a few feet to the tilt table and patting it, "why don't you let me help you?"

"Oh no, uh-uh," he said, shaking his head.

"Aw, come on," I chided. "I'll take it slow and easy and I'll stop when you say."

He considered it for a moment.

"Come on, hop up here," I said, patting the table.

"Okay," he conceded wearily. "But if I tell you to hold it,

115

you damned well better hold it," he added, stretching out on the table.

"I will. I will," I said absently as I searched under the table.

"What are you looking for?"

"A washcloth. I thought you might—"

"Well, I don't," he growled indignantly.

"Okay." I snickered. "But there are two ways to go about this—slow and easy or fast and funny."

"You're really enjoying this, aren't you?"

"Certainly not! I'm trying to show a little compassion. I'm trying to help another human being, a fellow traveler on the road of—"

"Never mind all that—just get on with it."

I slid a hand beneath Stirewalt's knee and raised it slightly, checking the weight of the massive leg.

"Easy, easy, easy, hold it, *hold it,*" he shouted.

"I haven't done anything yet."

"I know. I just wanted to remind you that we've got mat exercises coming up. You might want to keep that in mind."

"Ingrate! I'm trying to help you, and what do I get? Threats."

"Exactly." Stirewalt grinned.

Without averting my eyes, I reached out for his ankle and in one swift move flexed his knee to its limit. The ensuing roar rumbled through the gym like a clap of thunder.

"Ooooh, God. Ooooh, damn. You've ruined me!"

"I didn't ruin you. I cured you. Rise and walk."

"I can't. I can't straighten my leg," he moaned, easing his leg off the edge of the table and sitting up.

"See if you can stand on it."

"How can I stand on it if I can't straighten it. Get over there to the mats," he ordered, holding his knee with both hands.

"Are you sure you can't stand?"

"Not right now. Not for a few minutes."

"You're sure? You're sure you can't walk?"

"I'm sure!" he snapped.

"Well, I'll see ya," I said, grabbing the canes and heading for the door.

"Come back here! Don't you leave this gym!" he demanded.

Without answering, I hurried out of the gym and down the hall to hydrotherapy. "Harry, you got anybody scheduled for the Hubbard tank this hour?" I asked the attendant.

"Nope. Not until two thirty."

"You mind if I go ahead and take my treatment now?"

"You're not scheduled till four o'clock."

"I know, but I'm awful stiff."

"Well, it's all right with me. I guess it'll be okay."

Harry was reading a magazine a few minutes later when Stirewalt stuck his head in the door. "Did you see Helms come by here in the last few minutes?" he asked.

Without looking up, Harry jerked his thumb in the direction of the huge aluminum tank across the room. Stirewalt limped over and peered down into it. The only thing visible above the churning, bubbling water was my head, held afloat by an inflated rubber pillow.

"What the hell are you doing in there?" he bellowed. "Get the hell outta there."

"I can't get out. I've got to stay in here for at least thirty minutes."

"I'll wait."

"You can't wait. You've got clinic in twenty minutes and you'll be tied up in there all afternoon," I said with a superior smirk.

"You lizard! You goddamn lizard!" he grumbled helplessly. Then a smile flickered across his face.

I looked at him with a wary eye. "What are you going to do?" I asked cautiously. "Wait a minute now. Hold it!"

He reached down and pulled the plug from the pillow supporting my head and escaping air began to hiss by my ear.

"Don't do that!" I cried with alarm. "Put that back!"

He grinned down at me and then walked away, out of my range of vision.

"Stirewalt, come back here. You can't do that. I'll drown."

I heard the door open. I tried to reach the top of the tank but I couldn't get a grip on it. The door closed.

"Stirewalt! Stirewalt, you bastard. Harry? Harry, are you in here?" I shouted.

There was no answer, only the sound of the whirlpool and the steady hiss of air as the pillow slowly collapsed.

Harry was just dumb enough to let me drown, I thought as the swirling water reached my ears and began to erase all sound.

"Harry," I shouted, "if I drown there's going to be a scandal. A scandal, Harry. And they'll know I wasn't supposed to be in here and your ass'll be in the wringer. Harry—" Water boiled over in my mouth and I had to spit to keep from choking.

The pillow was almost gone, and it was all I could do to keep my nose above water when Harry grinned over the edge of the tank.

"Dumbass," I tried to say, but water filled my mouth and washed away the sound.

10

IT was several weeks later, on a Sunday, that I said good-bye to my family after an enjoyable evening and crossed the lobby on the way back to my room. It was almost nine o'clock and visiting hours would soon be over. I needed only one cane now and used it sparingly to correct a sense of balance that at times mysteriously failed me. My rhythmic steps were slow and deliberate, but my walking pattern was flawless. It would only be a matter of time and practice until the gait would once again consist of long graceful strides. I enjoyed walking as never before, the feel of my legs beneath me, the gentle sway of my body as the weight shifted effortlessly from one leg to the other, and the sound of it—the sound of my feet beating out a steady rhythm on the checkered tile floor, still slow, but a steady, constant sound that had cadence. It was no longer the shuffling, dragging sound it had been when I used the crutches, or the stumbling, capricious patter that had accompanied an awkward dependence on two canes. I had worked hard for that sound, and it had become a tocsin alerting me to the slightest variance in pattern.

119

Entering the room, I hooked the cane in the edge of an open drawer of the bedside cabinet and stretched out on the bed. I unsnapped the collar and tossed it on the cabinet, folded my hands behind my head, and stared thoughtfully at the ceiling. I would be going home in a few days. It would be a relief to get away from hospital schedules and hospital food. I was looking forward to home-cooked food and sleeping in my own bed. Just sleeping. It was going to be great to sleep late again, not to have some nurse poking a damp cloth in my face at seven o'clock every morning, announcing breakfast. To be able to come and go as I wanted, without having to be anywhere at a given time. Just to have some time of my own to while away frivolously, free of the nagging guilt of wasting precious minutes that could be put to use in the gym. And driving. To be able to get into a car and go somewhere, anywhere. I wondered if I would have any fear the first time I sat behind the wheel. Probably not. The accident didn't bother me that much—at least thinking about it or talking about it didn't. But what had started out to be a four-hour trip had taken almost seven months to complete.

It would be wonderful to be alone with myself once in a while. Since coming to Charlotte, I had not enjoyed a moment's privacy. There were times I needed solitude, longed for it. But it was going to be even more wonderful to be alone with a girl. I had been thinking about that a lot lately. Old needs were beginning to awaken. I was beginning to see the nurses differently—the way they moved, the way their perfume hung in the air after they left the room. It would certainly be good to have a date again.

I was wondering which girl I would call first when Glen's father, J.B., burst excitedly into the room and loudly announced that our suffering was at an end. He was a small, thin man with stooped shoulders, and his movements were quick and jerky. The old black suit coat he wore was threadbare and stained, with a ragged hole at one elbow, and his denim pants

120

were worn thin at the knee and seat. His leathery face was as eroded and weatherbeaten as the land he attempted to farm, but his eyes were shining with excitement.

"I'm on the Jesus road," he cried. "I've felt the sweet breath of Jesus."

I had seen J.B. many times but had talked to him only once. J.B. had become very agitated when I declined his offer to transport me by stretcher to a tent revival at which he had witnessed miraculous acts of healing. He had become even more outraged when he failed to secure permission to take his own son. I had avoided any further conversation with him for fear of triggering another outburst. J. B. Teeter was a man of mercurial responses which vacillated rapidly across a broad spectrum of emotion.

I watched with amusement now as he jerked the sheet off Glen's face while excitedly recounting an event at the evening prayer meeting.

"Folks was a glory-shoutin' an' talkin' in tongues," he said, pacing rapidly back and forth, gesturing wildly. "I was full up a grace an' full a the Holy Sperit an' that's when it come to me. I'd tried to figger her, Lord knows, I tried hard. I'd prayed an' prayed but it didn't do no good, an' the reason it didn't do no good was 'cause my idears was wrong. It ain't got nothin' to do with sin. You ain't done no wrong. Leastwise no big wrong. And it ain't got nothin' to do with punishment. Don't ya see, there's where I had her figgered wrong," he said to Glen in a voice cracking with dismay.

Glen ignored him, not bothering to look up from the TV. J.B. turned a pleading look toward me. "The Lord don't want you boys to suffer," he explained. "I thought He did an' that's somepin I worried over till I couldn't sleep at night. I jist couldn't figger the why of it. Then tonight it come clear to me for the first time. It was then that I knowed it weren't God that were doin' it. It's man! It's man what's interfered with God's plan an' caused all this sufferin' and pain. An' there 'neath the sweet breath of Jesus I knowed it was restin' with me to set it right," he said as he dug a bony hand into the pocket of his coat and fished around thoughtfully.

I nodded with a tired, conciliating smile and waited for him to retrieve a battered Bible which I knew would be waved about, pounded, thumped, and shaken in my face, as it had been so many times in Asheville. I hated that part of myself that was an open door to the needs of others, that part I could not control. It was not my responsibility to placate this old man any more than it had been my obligation to listen to the medical histories of almost everyone in the hospital. I would not allow myself the luxury of even a few minutes away from the gym or the exercises, but it was impossible for me to turn away from their tugging pleas, from the faint, brief cries of loneliness in their eyes. So I listened. And now I was about to be "saved" again. Damn Glen. Damn him for being able to do what I could not do.

J.B. tugged irritably at his pocket, clearing his hand just as Glen glanced up from the TV. He stared blankly for a moment before it registered. Then his face twisted in horrified disbelief.

"Oh, my God," I gasped when I saw the gun.

J.B. looked at me helplessly. "It's God's will."

"Now wait a minute, J.B., listen to me," I pleaded, reaching for the call buzzer. It was on the floor, out of reach.

"The Lord don't want you to suffer," he insisted.

"I'm not! I'm not suffering. I'm getting better," I said excitedly. "I'm going home in a few days."

"I seen ya. I seen how ya have ta use them sticks and yer legs shake and that thing you hafta wear on yer neck."

"That was a long time ago, J.B.," I pleaded. "My legs don't shake anymore, and I only use one cane now."

"Ya ain't never gonna be a whole man. I seen ya. An' it ain't right. The Lord didn't mean for that to happen. He was callin' you boys home till man got in the way of it," he said, taking a step toward me. "A man what breaks his neck ain't meant to live."

"Wait a minute, J.B., this is wrong," I said, fighting to keep the panic from my voice.

"It ain't wrong. It's the will of God."

"That's right, J.B.," Bo said suddenly. "You've been chosen to do the Lord's bidding and it would be a sin to—"

"Bo, you dirty son-of-a-bitch," I hissed. "You want to die so bad you don't care who you take with you. Just shut up! Shut your goddamn mouth!"

Bo must have seen something in my face because he reacted as though he'd been hit by a physical blow. His mouth hung there, open, silent.

J.B. was standing beside me. "It's what the Lord intended."

"Who the hell are you to—" I snapped and stopped in mid-sentence. Lose your temper and you're dead, I warned myself. Stay calm. And for God's sake—*think*.

J.B.'s arm came up swiftly and pressed the barrel of the gun tight against my temple. I wanted to scream. I was going to die! After all this I was going to die. I wanted to run, to hide, to be someone else, somewhere else. This wasn't happening—not to me. I heard the distinct double click of the pistol being cocked. My stomach knotted violently, sending waves of nausea through me. I was going to vomit. I was going to die and I was going to vomit and they were going to find me in a pool of blood and vomit. I had to stop this. I had to think. My mind raced wildly, frantically skimming the edges of a thousand fragmented thoughts, flashes of memory, emotion, fear. Hysteria! Don't panic, you bastard, I thought viciously. *Think!*

"I'm a sinner!" I cried, hoping it would not startle him into pulling the trigger. "Pray for me," I pleaded, looking up at him with all the innocence I could summon. "Don't send me to meet my maker stained with sin. Please, J.B., I've been a terrible sinner and I'm scared to die."

He looked down at me sympathetically. "Don't have no fear. The Lord'll forgive you."

"Ask the Lord to forgive me, J.B. He'll listen to you. He picked you to do his work, didn't He?"

123

He nodded and looked appraisingly at me. "I'll ast Him. I'll ast Him to have mercy on yer soul," he said, and without moving the pistol he began to pray.

I watched him cautiously and waited. When he had been praying for a few moments, watching closely for any reaction, I softly said, "Praise be." He did not seem to notice. Taking care not to break the rhythm of the prayer, I raised my voice slightly and added, "Amen." He did not notice. As the fervor of his prayer intensified, I continued to punctuate it with "amens" and "glory be's," getting louder with each one. J.B., oblivious to everything except his prayer, let his voice rise with mine.

I was shouting at the top of my voice when the nurse finally came. Her angry strides carried her several feet into the room before she gasped in horror and froze, staring with terrified incredulity at J.B., lost in the feral howl of his prayer, and at me, a pistol pressed to my head, screaming "HALLELUJAH, GOD HAVE MERCY!"

Looking beyond J.B., I saw the nurse back slowly out of the room and disappear down the hall. I watched the door and continued to punctuate and prolong J.B.'s prayer for long, endless seconds until the nurse finally returned with a guard who approached J.B. from behind, noiselessly.

I felt a wild, rampant panic seize me when the guard hesitated and seemed undecided as to what course of action to take. Then in a single move the guard wrapped a huge arm around J.B.'s throat, jerked his head back, and snatched the pistol from his hand.

I closed my eyes, inhaled deeply, and let the breath out slowly as my weight sank heavily into the bed. Never had I been so tired.

"You selfish son-of-a-bitch," I heard Bo say after they had taken J.B. away. "That was my ticket out of here. He wouldn't have gotten off more than one shot before that guard would have been in here. But you don't care, do you? You're getting out."

124

I wondered why Bo thought that one shot would have been for him when the gun was pointed at me. I started to ask him. I started to ask him if it wasn't possible that after that first shot the guard might have had to shoot it out with J.B., but I didn't. I didn't say anything. I didn't even open my eyes.

The following Wednesday Stirewalt and I stood in front of the hospital waiting for my father to bring the car around from the parking lot. I found it an altogether strange feeling to be outside the protective environment of the hospital after such a long time.

"The wind's got a little bite to it, but other than that it's a beautiful day," Stirewalt said.

"Yes, it is," I answered and was struck by how unchanged it all was. Nothing had changed. I had expected it to be different somehow.

"You got that list of exercises I gave you?" he asked.

"Yeah, in my bag."

"And you'll do them every day?"

"Yes, you know I will."

"Well, don't push it. Don't punish your legs. And don't try to get rid of the cane too soon."

"Okay."

"I want you to carry it for the next couple of months at least. Carry it until it's a damn nuisance. Carry it until you don't use it."

"Okay."

"Wait until you're getting around without it real well inside before you try going outside without it."

"Okay."

"And watch it around loose gravel and on steps until your balance improves."

"All right. All right." I laughed.

"I mean it. You can't afford a fall, not yet. How long does Walters want you to wear the collar?"

"Another six months."

"Good. I was afraid he was going to take you out of it too soon. Well, I guess that's it then. Any questions you want to ask me?"

"No, nothing I can think of."

There was an awkward silence. He stared speculatively at me for a moment, seemed about to say something, then looked down at the pavement. He glanced restlessly toward the parking lot, then back at me. "Well, hard nose," he said, extending his huge hand, "take care and stay in touch. Let us hear from you."

"Yeah, I will," I said, my hand swallowed up by his. I hesitated for a moment. "I don't know how to begin to—"

"Uh-uh, no," he protested, shaking his head and averting his eyes. Then he shrugged. "Just doing my job." He released my hand and started for the door. He stopped and looked back at me. "You're a champion, a goddamn champion." Then he disappeared into the hospital.

I stared after him for a moment and felt the loss. I was going to miss him. Looking toward the parking lot, I noticed the fall colors and felt it again—the sameness. Something should have changed. It should look different. I should see it differently, I thought. Wasn't an experience like mine supposed to bring with it a new awareness, a wisdom born of pain? The only thing pain had taught me was an understanding of pain. It hadn't opened any doors or revealed any secrets.

The brisk autumn wind snatched at my hair, sending a shiver through me, and I was suddenly aware of the warmth within me—and the loneliness.

11

I had come to the gym looking for a fraternity brother and I was glad that was all I was looking for because the gym was a madhouse. More than ten thousand students were trying to register for classes that were already closed out, canceled or full. The line stretched across the stadium parking lot, doubled back on itself at the football field, came back by the gym, and snaked up Lumpkin Street. You could almost smell the confusion and feel the anger in the rumble of the overheated, overcrowded gym.

I had sworn I would never go through registration again—not after the first time. I had made that mistake when I first came to the University of Georgia two years earlier. It was at the beginning of my sophomore year and I had decided then that there had to be a better way of getting the classes I needed. I would have found a way of doing it on my own if the necessity hadn't been removed when I joined a fraternity that had a member who knew someone in the registrar's office.

I glanced over my shoulder in the direction of the moans and mumbled obscenities that greeted a sign announcing the closing of another class and walked into her, almost knocking her off her feet. Class cards, tuition cards, health cards, fee cards, envelopes, announcement bulletins, and special marking pencils flew in all directions.

"Why don't you watch where you're going," she yelled in a voice quavering with exasperation. "Of all the stupid—that's all I need. The end of a perfect day."

"I'm sorry," I shouted above the roar.

She was saying something, but I couldn't hear her above the noise. I wouldn't have heard her if we had been alone in an empty gym. She was the most beautiful girl I'd ever seen.

She was tall, with long blond hair that curved in and nestled against the lightly tanned skin of her face. Frustration and anger flashed from enormous black-lashed blue-green eyes. She stood with her shoulders pulled back, her full, round breasts thrust defiantly forward. Her mouth was full-lipped and soft. As she looked down at the scattered cards which were being walked on and kicked about by the pressing mass of students, her face darkened with resignation.

"You're going to pick that up," she announced, pointing a finger at the floor.

"Look, I said I was sorry. Just calm down," I said, trying to restrain a grin.

With a coldly accusing stare, she spread her long, trim legs, planted both hands firmly on hips that flared out beautifully below an incredibly small waist, and pressed her lips into a tight, straight line.

"Pick it up."

I looked expressionlessly at her for a moment, then I spread my legs, put my hands on my hips, pressed my lips together in an exaggerated scowl and, doing my best to imitate her glaring look, leaned forward bringing my face down to hers. My nose was almost touching hers when I said, "I ain't sure, but I think I can whip you."

She took in a quick deep breath, her chin jutted forward, the stare turned to ice. Then she let the air out, her eyes softened, and her shoulders rolled forward as she broke into a broad smile.

"I'm sorry. I guess I was just looking for somebody to take it out on. This day has been . . ." She let the sentence drop and slowly shook her head.

"What seems to be the problem?—other than people trying to walk over you, I mean," I asked as we stooped and began picking up the cards.

"This." She gestured toward students clamoring around tables set at right angles to each other like small forts across the gym. "This whole incredible mess. There ought to be a better way. There's got to be a better way. Would you believe I've been here for four hours—four solid hours! And now they tell me poly sci one-oh-five is closed out." She shook her head again.

"So rearrange your schedule."

She looked at me slowly as though she couldn't believe I had said it.

"Okay, so pick it up next quarter. Take something else this term."

"I wish it were that simple."

"It is."

"It is not. This is the only time I have room for it. The classes offered winter and spring quarters are a must, and they are offered *only* during winter and spring terms. This isn't mine," she said, handing me a card I had just picked up for her.

"You're sure?" I mused, looking at the name on the card and standing up. "You're sure you aren't Jefferson Allen Shropshire?"

"You can joke. You're not closed out of the one class you've got to have."

"And you aren't either," I said seriously. "Not if that one class is all you need. I can get you in."

She looked at me with probing distrust.

"I've got a system."

"Oh, sure. Great. Fine."

"No, really."

"Look around, there must be six or seven thousand people in here, and every one of them has a system that will beat the system and not one—*not one*—works."

"Well, it's obvious that you don't recognize genius when it runs into you. I ought to leave you here—"

"Please do. It would be the first thing that's gone right all day."

"You're getting hostile again, but fortunately I was raised among the hostiles. I'm not offended. I come in peace. I don't want your land or your women. I only want to lead you out of darkness and ignorance and into political science one-oh-five."

"You're crazy."

"Of course I'm crazy. Earth's the loony bin of the universe, and this is the violent ward. Come on, I'll buy you a cup of coffee and tell you how to get in that class."

She was hesitant.

"What have you got to lose? If it's closed out, it's closed out, and you're never going to get it hanging around this nut farm," I said, taking her by the arm and heading her toward the door.

The waitress set the coffee on the table, half spilling it, and hurried off.

"I'm Cory Benton," she said, and her short straight nose wrinkled when she smiled.

"I'm Tom Helms," I told her, and I thought I had never seen a face more perfect. It needed no assistance, and the little color she had added to her lips made them appear ready to burst. I had to restrain myself from reaching out to touch that face.

"So tell me, how do I do it?"

"Simple, you just walk in and sit down."

"I'm going to get up and walk out is what I'm going to do."

"Why does it have to be complicated? If I offered you an intricate scheme, you'd go for it in a second. I'm offering you a simple solution to a simple problem, and you better be glad I'm keeping it simple because it's beginning to look like I don't have much to work with."

"Well, what can you expect from an ignorant savage living in darkness?"

"Drink your coffee, Pocahontas, and listen. First of all, a student picks up a computer card at registration, which is what you were unable to do, gives it to the professor the first day of class. Now, he lays it on his desk and passes around a seating chart for everybody to sign—that is, if he gives a damn whether or not you attend class. He won't make a seating chart from the cards the way he should. Oh, no, that's clerical work, and never forget he considers himself an intellectual—far above that sort of thing.

"Now, after class he sends the cards to Administration for a computer printout, which will be the official roll and will take about ten days to come back. In the meantime, if he checks attendance at all, he will use the seating chart—which, of course, you're on. During those ten days be sure he notices you. Answer questions. Ask questions. Then when the official roll comes back, act bewildered because your name isn't on it. He'll think it's a computer mistake and send in a card to have your name added. Simple."

She looked at me with an uncertain grin. "You're serious."

"You bet your sweet feathers I'm serious."

"What if there are just so many seats in the class and a card has been issued for each one?"

"There's always somebody that doesn't show. But get there early just in case, and if somebody's left standing the professor'll think one too many cards were printed. At any rate, he won't waste time trying to figure it out—that's clerical—he won't do it. These guys have got a real thing about intellectual freedom and not getting bogged down in the mechanics of it all.

131

They consider anything Administration asks them to do as an assault on their personal rights as free thinkers."

"You know, it just might work," she said, staring at me with a big, fascinated grin.

"It's not easy, this life I've chosen for myself. It's full of unending days and lonely nights—hardships and deprivation. But when I can reach out and take a heathen by the hand and lead her into light—when I can look into the smiling face of a grateful convert as I'm looking into yours now—well, I tell you, it's worth it."

Cory Benton laughed, and her voice was rich and low and full of music. Then we sat silently. She studied my face and her eyes darkened. At that moment I felt as if I had come home after a long absence.

"Tell me about Tom Helms," she said.

"There really isn't very much to tell."

"Well, for starters, how'd you get that little scar on the bridge of your nose?"

"Would you believe," I said, running a finger across my nose, "that this is the result of underestimating a guy with the unlikely nickname of Peachy?"

Three hours later I glanced at my watch and was surprised by the time.

"Good Lord, girl, do you realize I've been rambling on for almost three hours? You should have stopped me."

She shook her head. "I've enjoyed it. Maybe I was caught up in the fervor of a new convert."

"Well, it is getting late, why don't we grab a bite to eat and stop by Allen's. If we're lucky, we might even get a table."

"I'm sorry, I have plans for this evening."

My heart sank. But she sounded sincere, I thought. Her voice was tinged with real regret.

"Tomorrow then. We could have dinner at the fraternity house and stick around for the party. There's a great combo coming over from Atlanta. And besides, I feel I should keep

132

an eye on you. I wouldn't want you slipping back into your heathen ways."

"Well, as long as it's purely professional I suppose it will be all right." She smiled. "It sounds like fun. I'd love to."

I picked her up at eight the next evening and she was even lovelier than I remembered. She was dressed in a simple white skirt and a blue blouse and was wearing her hair pulled back, exposing a beautifully delicate neck.

The party was perfect except that there were people there, as there had been at the gym and at the coffee shop, and I had no interest in people or parties. I had no interest in dancing either; usually it bored me but tonight it was different, especially when the evening grew late and the music slowed, becoming soft and mellow with the time and the mood and she no longer danced several feet away from me but moved her body with mine, against mine. She nestled her face against my neck and moved with me like she was part of me.

"This is nice," she said and her breath against my neck sent a current coursing through me.

I shifted her away from me slightly and looked down at her. She met the look and we danced that way for what seemed forever. I started to pull her to me, to kiss her. It would have been natural, it would have been what the moment demanded. But then I remembered the people around us. I had forgotten them, and normally they wouldn't have bothered me. They never had before. But this was different, Cory Benton was different, my feelings were different, and those feelings weren't to be shared with those around us, they weren't to be displayed on a dance floor.

I started to suggest going by my apartment for a drink, but I decided against it. Here the situation called for a kiss and that, for her, might be all it called for. The mood was here, it was now, and it might not be recaptured at my apartment. Going there would suggest more. You don't need to go to an apartment for a kiss. Maybe somewhere on the way back to the dorm. Maybe we could stop somewhere on campus— I almost laughed. I couldn't believe it. Me plotting a kiss, a simple kiss. There had been a hundred girls and I had never thought about what to do, or when, or where. I did what I felt like when I felt like it, and if it turned out wrong, so what. You didn't work at these things. Why? Why put forth any effort? To end up lying in bed staring at the ceiling and wondering why in hell you went to all the trouble. To have to hold someone when you no longer felt like holding her. To have to talk and stroke and be attentive, when the only feeling you had was one of disgust for yourself for plotting and lying and scheming and not saying what you felt like saying when you felt like saying it because the truth would keep her from your bed.

"Well, it is nice, isn't it?" she asked.

I smiled at her. "Yes, it's nice and I'm glad you decided to come."

I pulled her to me, her face against my neck and I held her tighter. I wasn't plotting a simple kiss. I wasn't plotting anything. I just wanted to do what seemed to be the most natural thing in the world, only I wanted to do it in private and I was trying to figure out where to find that privacy.

We continued dancing, holding each other, moving as one, not saying anything and saying everything.

"Let's walk back instead of driving," I finally suggested.

"All right."

"It's a long walk, you're sure you don't mind?"

"I'm sure. Some fresh air would be welcome right now."

She spoke softly as we walked, telling me about herself, about her family or lack of family. She was an only child and her father had left them shortly after she was born. She had never known her father, and there had never been any word from him.

The night air of early fall was warm and heavy and scent-filled. Frail moonlight filtering through ancient oaks spread an intricate mantle of lace over deserted paths.

134

We moved around a fallen branch and she brushed against me. I reached for her, pulled her to me, and her face turned, moving up to meet mine. I pressed her to me and felt the softness and warmth of her. Her lips responded to mine, her body strained at me and lingered for endless moments. I felt in myself an urgency I had never known. There was a soft moan and she stepped back, away from me. She looked at me, into me, searching, then she was in my arms again.

We walked even more slowly after that, trying to make the night last, but all too soon we were at her dorm and there were people again.

She kissed me on the cheek. "Well, Thomas, it's—"

"How about the ball game tomorrow? Go with me?"

Her expression became one of regret. "I'm sorry. I have plans for tomorrow."

"So do I." I grinned. "But I'm going to change mine."

She looked at me for a moment, decided that I was serious, and considered it. Then she smiled mischievously. "Okay, I'll change my plans."

"Great. I'll pick you up at one."

We went to the game the next afternoon and then out to dinner, where we ran into friends of Cory's who insisted we join them for the evening. On Sunday we went for a long, quiet drive and when classes began on Monday I was delighted to find that our paths crossed following the last class of the day. We slipped into an easy routine of meeting after class, stopping to eat, and studying together in the evenings, always at the library or in one of the study rooms of her dorm. There was seldom any privacy, and no matter how well I presented the advantages, she found an excuse for not going to my apartment.

It had been two weeks to the day since we first met. I watched her hurrying toward me, waving a yellow card above her head.

"It worked," she yelled excitedly. "It worked. I'm in the

class—officially on the rolls." Balancing her books on her hip, she stretched up to kiss me. "Isn't that beautiful?"

"Yeah . . . sure," I said with a silly grin. "It really worked, eh?"

"Yes! It worked! I'm in. He cursed the computer and damned the system and called Admin—" She stepped back and looked at me soberly. A frown wrinkled her brow.

"It's not what you think," I said, shaking my head and backing away.

"You *rat!*"

"Now hold on—wait a minute."

"You dirty—"

"I can explain . . ."

"You never tried it. You didn't know if it would work."

"Well . . ." I shrugged helplessly.

"Of all the dirty, lowdown, despicable tricks," she said, reaching for a book.

"Now hold on! Hold it right there," I ordered, rising to my full height. "Don't you throw that book."

Cory's arm dropped to her side, the book dangling in her hand. Her stare was indignant as she measured me with her eyes.

"Now if you'll just listen—"

I ducked quickly to my right and the fluttering book narrowly missed my head.

"Wait a minute—"

"You wait a minute," she yelled. "How could you do such a thing? How could you let—"

"Just calm down. People are staring," I told her, nodding toward gathering students.

"Let 'em! They ought to stare. You're something to see—a real phenomenon—a two-legged louse."

"It worked, didn't it? That's all that matters. It worked. What are you getting so upset about?"

"I can't believe you did it," she said, shaking her head bit-

136

terly. "I can't believe you let me go into that class with some harebrained scheme—"

"Harebrained scheme! Harebrained scheme! Well, I like that. It was a well-thought-out plan—perfect. And I only had the few minutes between the gym and the coffee shop to come up with it. Besides, you had an ace going in—couldn't fail."

"What ace?" she asked scornfully.

"With a set of legs like that—no man in his right mind would throw you out of class." I grinned.

"You're a real genius, aren't you? Had it all covered, didn't you? Well, let's say you're right—and it would be the first time—what if the professor had been a woman? Huh? What then?"

"Well, I can't think of everything," I said, walking over to pick up the fallen book. When I offered it to her, she made no move to take it. She stood looking at me with astonishment.

"Look," I conceded, "I wouldn't have let you try it unless I was willing to do it myself. I wouldn't. I knew it would work, or at least I was sure enough that I would have tried it myself, and my legs aren't nearly as pretty as yours."

She smiled and shook her head with disbelief.

It rained the next day, and we were unprepared for it, except for a plastic bonnet she miraculously produced from the depths of an overstuffed purse. It started as a fine mist in the second quarter of the game, but by the fourth quarter the muddy players were barely visible through the downpour. We left before the game was over, but rather than walk to the fraternity house for dinner as we had planned, we decided to stop by my apartment so I could change into dry clothes and pick up my car. Then I could drive her to the dorm to change and go on to dinner from there.

When we entered the apartment I cursed myself for not keeping the place neater. The shirt I had picked up at the cleaner's two days earlier was draped over a chair, books and papers were piled on the dining room table, records and record jackets were strewn everywhere.

"Damn, I've been burglarized!" I said.

"How can you tell?" She laughed.

"We'll just have to make the best of it, I guess. Mix us a drink while I get into something dry," I said, pointing toward the kitchen.

I grimaced as I entered the bedroom. She would want to see the rest of the apartment, and I would hate for her to see this. I opened the top drawer of the dresser and raked everything off the dresser into it, kicked a pair of shoes under the bed, picked up several shirts and pairs of pants and threw them into the closet. I sat a half-empty cup of cold coffee in the medicine cabinet and straightened up the bathroom. Then I quickly changed into dry clothes.

Coming out of the bedroom I stopped. She was standing at the kitchen counter with her back to me. She was wearing only my shirt. I glanced at the chair where it had been and saw her clothes neatly hung over the heat vent.

"It's so bad out I thought we might fix something here rather than going out again," she said without turning around.

"Yeah, sure. That sounds fine," I said, and the words came out like broken glass, chipped and jagged and catching in my throat.

"Is this all you have?" she asked, turning from the cabinets to face me. The front of the shirt swayed with the movement of her breasts.

"No, there's some—" I caught myself. I was speaking too loudly, trying to make myself heard above the roar of my blood. I moved to the counter and opened another cabinet. "There's some more stuff up here."

I reached for a can on the lower shelf just as she reached across for one farther back. Her breast mashed against my arm—firm and warm and almost naked beneath the thin fabric of my shirt. I drew my arm down slowly across her breast and reached around her, turning her into me. I kissed her warm mouth deeply and felt her body quiver as she locked her arms around me. Without saying anything, I led her to the bedroom and, standing beside the bed, kissed her again. I unbuttoned the front of her shirt and slipped my hand in against silky skin. She made a soft moaning noise and twisted her body, bringing her soft, full breast into my hand. I slipped the shirt off her shoulders and let it fall to the floor. She fumbled with the buttons of my shirt and when I stepped back to remove it the breath caught in my throat at the sight of her.

I undressed quickly and gently pulled her onto the bed. I had my arms around her and her lips bit at my mouth. I rolled into her, pressing the full length of my body against her, crushing her to me. She strained against me violently and as I lifted myself over her she met me eagerly.

It was dark when I awoke to find her still asleep in the crook of my nearly paralyzed arm. I was pleased to find her there, and this particular pleasure was new to me. Always before, my need for women had been spent with my passion. I gently brushed the loose blond hair away from her face and wondered if I would ever get enough of her, if I would ever tire of just looking at that beautiful face and perfectly sculptured body.

But Cory Benton was more than that. She was a part of me. She made me whole. She had been the reason for my anger and my refusal to give up life. She was what death had tried to cheat me of, and I wondered if she would ever know that I was alive because of her, that she had given my life direction long before we met.

She stretched and yawned. When she opened her eyes, she smiled and snuggled closer to me.

"You love me, you know," she said.

"I know."

"I'm glad."

"I'm starving."

She giggled and propped up on one arm and looked down at me. She slowly ran a finger over my lips.

"You've got a beautiful mouth."

139

"I'm glad."

"I'm starving."

I laughed and she kissed me lightly on the lips.

"What's this?" she asked, touching the quarter-inch scar at the base of my throat.

"I was in an automobile accident once."

"Serious?"

"Uh-huh."

"You could have died?"

"I suppose. But I knew you were waiting somewhere down the road, and if I didn't show you'd wander around lost forever."

"That's true," she said seriously. "You didn't mean it, but it's true."

I looked at her. Then I pulled her down to me.

At Thanksgiving break Cory insisted that I go home to Savannah with her. I was looking forward to meeting her mother, whom I expected to be a mature replica of Cory, someone whose beauty had been enhanced by the years—and not too many years at that. I expected her to be in her early forties—blond, beautiful, confident, and poised. It would be a look into the future, a look at what the years held in store for Cory.

But Cory's mother was none of these things. She was old, and the years had not been kind. Bitterness was etched in the deep lines of her face. She was small and stooped and wore her thin, graying brown hair gathered in a loose, wispy knot at the back of her head. Cory had been an unwelcome burden that had come terribly late in life.

She did not smile when I was introduced to her, and if she had ever been beautiful there was no remnant of that beauty—not in her face and not in her soul. She made no attempt to hide her obvious displeasure that I was her guest for the weekend, and it soon became evident that I was not what she had in mind for her daughter. She considered Cory an investment.

Cory was beautiful, and there was a market for beauty. A market full of doctors and lawyers and the sons of rich men, and I was none of these.

It was a very long and unpleasant weekend.

"I wouldn't rate myself as one of your mother's all-time favorite people," I said to Cory on our drive back.

"She would be like that with anybody—any male—I brought home. I'm her little girl, remember?"

I did remember and I avoided going back.

Cory went home with me over the Christmas holidays, and Rick fell in love with her. He vowed to spend every weekend in Athens until we found him someone exactly like her, and if we failed at this, his only recourse would be to kill me, step in to console Cory, and win her heart in the process. Cory was crazy about him.

When spring break came, I could avoid it no longer. During the dreary months of winter we had talked often of getting away from the weather, of spending those few precious days of spring break on a warm sunny beach. I hadn't been thinking of Savannah Beach when we talked, but Cory had. "And besides," she argued, "why spend money we don't have to spend?" I couldn't argue with that, especially since money was becoming a problem, so I agreed and once again became her mother's guest. Once again the reception was cold, the extended weekend over-long, and the bitter months of winter took on a remembered warmth.

I began job interviews at the beginning of spring quarter and four weeks into the quarter I had my second offer. It was a management training position with a manufacturing firm in Knoxville, and it was better than anything I had expected. I walked out of the interview knowing I was going to accept the offer.

I stood looking over the parking lot, trying to locate my car, and I felt a sensation that was totally new to me. I was eight weeks away from graduation, I had a couple of good job offers, a girl, and a firm grip on the future, and there it was stretched out in front of me—life. Stretched out and ready to be lived. I could go anywhere I wanted, do anything I wanted. There wasn't one single thing left that I *had* to do. I was through preparing.

I had been in school for seventeen years, and for as long as I could remember I had worked during the summers. I went to school because it was necessary, not because I wanted to. I'd never really done anything I wanted to do. Well, now it was my turn. I'd been running one maze after another all my life—one narrow corridor after another—and suddenly I was going to be out. No more walls. No more long, confining corridors that *had* to be traveled. It was time to do what I wanted to, and I knew exactly what I wanted to do first.

I left my car and walked to the psychology building and waited. She would be getting out of class in a few minutes.

"How'd it go?" she asked when she saw me.

I held up a thumb and grinned.

"You got the job?" she squealed. "You really got it?" She dropped her books and threw her arms around my neck.

"I got it," I said as I swung her around in a circle. "I got it."

I put her down and stepped back and looked at her seriously. She noted the look and her expression became thoughtful as she studied my face.

"Marry me, Cory."

She just looked at me for a moment, then her expression changed to one of infinite wisdom. She smiled and looked at me as though I were a child who had just realized a truth that had been obvious forever.

"In June," she said, and her arms were around my neck.

I swung her in a wide circle and clasped her to me, enjoying the moment, the relief that she had said yes. Then what she had said sank in—exactly what she had said. I stopped and put her down.

"In June?" I asked, freeing myself from her embrace. "We don't graduate until June."

"The first of June. We can be married at the end of June."

I laughed. "I don't have any money. We can't get married in June."

"Yes we can."

"No we can't. Now listen, I've got to work a couple of months first. I think a fall wedding would be nice."

"Fall? That means we'll be apart all summer."

"Well, I don't see any other way to swing it. When I say I don't have any money, I mean *no money*. I'm flat busted. What I made last summer isn't even going to get me through this quarter."

She pouted while I picked up her books.

"Okay," she said, "August."

"August isn't fall." I laughed. "Fall is October—September maybe. Come on, you want to get something to eat?"

"No," she said, slipping her arm in mine and smiling at me mysteriously. "I want to go to your apartment. I think you have something to learn about the seasons."

Cory finally conceded that there was no way financially that we could get married before late September and she began making plans for the wedding and for the apartment we would have. Her mother objected vehemently and more than once a telephone call from her left Cory in tears. But we went ahead with our plans and decided to have a small wedding in a chapel in Savannah; that way we wouldn't have to ask for any financial help from anyone. Cory insisted on paying for it herself.

My family was delighted, and when they came down the day before graduation they exuberantly welcomed Cory into the family. Her mother arrived later in the day and we took them out to dinner. The atmosphere was strained, as I expected it to be, but what I had not expected was Cory's silence. She hardly spoke at all during the meal and when I tried to catch her eye she looked away.

We dropped her mother at her motel and my family at theirs. Thank God they had selected different motels, I thought.

"Okay, you want to tell me what's wrong," I asked as we drove away from the motel. She didn't answer. "Bad scene with your mother this afternoon?" I asked.

She exhaled slowly. "Yes, I guess you could call it that."

"Want to talk about it?"

She didn't answer immediately. Then she said, "How would you feel about waiting a year before we get married?"

I thought she was kidding. I thought she was referring to how long the wait until September seemed to both of us.

"Not too good," I said.

"Well, that's what she wants us to do."

I looked at her and there were tears running down her face. I had never seen anyone look so helpless.

"Why? What would that accomplish?"

"Nothing probably, but she says she wants me to be on my own for at least a year before I get married. Experience, you know. Invaluable, they say." Her tone was flat, edged with bitterness.

"And what did you say?"

"What could I say?"

"No, I hope."

"Tom, she's not telling me not to do something. She's not even asking me *not* to marry you. She's asking me to do something for her—that's the way she put it—for her. She's never asked me to do anything for her, and now she's asking."

"You're not seriously considering waiting, are you?"

She didn't answer, and when I looked at her she was staring into the floor of the car, her chin set slightly forward. I knew that stubborn look and I knew that she had made her decision and no amount of argument from me could change it, but I was damn well going to try. I couldn't believe that this could happen, that her mother could pull from her arsenal a weapon so unexpectedly devastating.

144

"Cory, you see what she's doing, don't you?"

"Yes, I know what she's doing."

"She's buying time. She's stalling. Give her a year, and at the end of that time she'll have another reason. She'll ask for something else."

"Don't you think I know that," she snapped. "Don't you think I know exactly what she's doing. But, Tom, I owe her something."

"Of course you owe her. We all owe our parents and we pay them in whatever coin we can, but this . . . this isn't payment of anything."

"It's granting her the first and only thing she's ever asked of me."

"But her reasons. Don't her reasons count?"

"No."

I thought about waiting a year and found myself looking down another long, empty corridor, running another maze, and another and another, and for what? My anger flared.

"I'll be goddamned if I'm going to let her do this, if I'm going to let them do this." I spat the words at her. "I'm tired, Cory—I'm goddamn tired of living my life for other people, for the things they want, for the things they think are important. I've got a life! When do you think I can start living it?"

"Tom, a year isn't so long—"

"Yes it is. Yesterday you thought three months were going to be unbearable, and now a year isn't so long?"

I pulled the car into the dormitory parking lot, switched off the motor, and sat there.

"What are you going to do?" she asked when it became evident that I had no more to say.

"I'm going to Knoxville, I'm going to start a new job, and I'm going to do what's right for me."

"And what's right for you isn't giving up another year of your life for my mother, huh?"

"Cory, I'd wait a year or five years or however long it takes

145

if it was necessary, if it served some purpose, but this is foolish."

"I know," she said softly. "I know you would. And I know this is foolish, but damn it, Tom, she's given up a lot for me. It wasn't easy bringing me up alone, and now to deny her the first thing she asks."

"Will it be any easier the second time?" I asked bitterly.

She didn't answer me.

"Cory, I know I'm being a bastard about this—I know what you're up against, and I know I'm sticking you right in the middle. I'm making you choose, but it's going to come to that eventually—the day's going to come—so why not now?"

"Because it's the first time. I knew the day I met you that that day was coming. I also know that we love each other and I think you'll give me this—when you have time to think about it."

"And I think that once you realize I'm not, you'll tell your mother you'll make payment some other way."

"I hope to God only one of us is wrong, because if we both are . . ."

She didn't finish the sentence. She stepped out of the car and walked off toward the dorm.

As I drove back to my apartment I still couldn't believe it would happen. Once she realized I was serious she'd come around. Her mother had her in a bind. She didn't want to wait and she wouldn't throw away something she wanted by doing something she didn't want to do—first time or no damn first time.

I didn't see her during graduation exercises and I didn't call her afterwards. I didn't have anything more to say and, if she didn't hear from me in a few days, she'd realize how serious I was.

My parents left for home and my brother stayed, helping me load the car. It took longer than we expected and it was late when we finally pulled out of Athens. I didn't feel any sense of loss because I was sure I would hear from her.

146

It was late when we reached home. My parents were already in bed, so we decided to wait until morning to unload the car.

When I awoke it was early. No one was up yet, and I cursed under my breath for not having brought in the suitcase with my jeans in it. All I had was the dress pants I had worn home. I pulled them on and went out to the car.

As I pulled the huge suitcase out from the boxes and other bags in the trunk, I swore aloud and wondered what I had managed to squeeze into it that weighed so much.

As I lugged it up the steps I had to lean awkwardly to the left to counterbalance the weight of the oversized monster.

I wondered if Cory would call today. Probably not. It was too soon. I had to be in Knoxville in a week. Maybe she would call before then, but I didn't really think so. She was stubborn; it would take a while. I'd call her, but that wouldn't accomplish anything, and it might convince her that sooner or later I'd give her that year. I'd just have to wait it out—she'd call.

Just as I reached the top step the handle on the old suitcase snapped with the report of a gunshot and the suitcase fell away. I was overbalanced and fell backwards to the left. Hoping to break the fall with my hands, I spun around just in time to reach for the rear bumper of the car, but it was wet with early morning dew and my hand slipped. The bumper caught me just above the left eye, driving my head back.

12

A *benevolent breeze was sweeping away the fog, and the humming in my head was blending into a steady pounding. I wasn't hung over and I wasn't dreaming and the nightmare wasn't going to go away. I had to move something. I had to move a toe, only I didn't want to try.* I couldn't remember riding. *Maybe I wasn't in Asheville. I could remember insisting that they bring me, insisting against all protest. Move the toe. Yes, I was in Asheville. Mom would have seen to that. She had promised. It was in the emergency room just before I lost consciousness. Yes, I was in Asheville and McKinnon had operated. I could remember seeing him. Now all I had to do was move something. But why couldn't I remember riding? I had passed out, sure, but I had been coming and going and passing out all over the place. I braced against a sudden surge of pain. I let my breath out slowly and relaxed the tensed muscles of my jaw. I didn't want to try to move my toe. I didn't want to try to move anything. I wanted to be normal and as long as I didn't try, as long as I could ignore the pain, I was normal. But I couldn't ignore the pain and I couldn't clear my head and I couldn't hide forever. So, I would move a toe.*

My heart almost stopped—it moved! *My toe moved! I felt like laughing and singing and yelling. By God, it moved. I could even rotate my foot. I couldn't feel it, but it moved, it responded. All I had to do was tell it to move and, by God, it moved—my whole foot moved. But that was all that moved. The leg was dead and I felt sick. Sicker than I had ever felt. I couldn't bend my knee. I tried. Again and again I tried. I couldn't get any response from my leg—either leg. I tried again. I tried with all my strength to bend my knee and, as I did, the fingers of my right hand curled into a fist. I couldn't feel it. It was numb but it moved. Sensory nerves. McKinnon had explained it once. Sensory nerves and motor nerves. What had he said? I couldn't remember. I couldn't clear the dulling fog out of my head.*

I brought my fist up, inch by creeping inch, until my forearm pointed toward the ceiling. I began to straighten a trembling arm, reaching for the ceiling, but the effort was too much. My arm fell. I tried the fingers of my left hand. Nothing.

So that was it, I thought bitterly. Goddammit, it wasn't fair. There ought to be some kind of justice. It just wasn't fair. One foot. One lousy damn foot and my right arm. What kind of justice was that? I couldn't do it again. I wasn't that brave. I wasn't that stupid. I wasn't a naïve kid anymore. I knew what lay ahead. I knew! I knew!

I could feel myself beginning to slip. There was something missing. Something I had had before. I felt completely defenseless. I couldn't go through it again. I had read something once about the gods testing the ones they loved. Was it "loved" or "chosen"? Those chosen by the gods are sorely tried? Those loved *by the gods are sorely tried. Either way it didn't make much sense. It was stupid. Goddamn stupid rhetoric spouted by some* un*loved son-of-a-bitch. I wished I was unloved—unloved and untried. The gods could play their game with somebody else. It wasn't fair. I wasn't a game. I shouldn't be rolled like so many dice. I shouldn't be broken while they sat around* on some far-off Olympus and bet on which way I would fall. A black anger rose in me. Now I had found what had been missing. I picked up my weapon.

When next I was conscious of anything it was a drum being pounded somewhere in the back of my head and a cool, damp cloth being pressed to my forehead. I must have asked for the cloth. I could remember something being said about a cloth but that was days ago. Or was it?

"Hi. I believe you drifted off again," Mom said when I opened my eyes.

"What—" My lips began to crack. I ran the tip of my tongue over them and tried again. "What time is it?"

"Two o'clock," she said, then noticing the look, quickly added, "in the afternoon."

"Of the same day?"

"The same day as what?"

"The same day I asked for that cloth."

"Yes." She laughed. "It's the same day you asked for the cloth."

Well, that straightened that out, I thought, and it was a relief to get something straightened out at last, except I didn't have the vaguest idea of what I had straightened out. Each beat of my heart was a hammer blow to the back of my head, blurring my vision and sending stabbing pains down my neck.

"My head feels like it's gonna explode."

"Yes, I know. They'd give you something—a shot. But you told me never to let them give you a shot."

"Never *let 'em give me a shot*."

"Maybe it won't make you sick like it did before."

"It'll make me sick and I'll die."

"You won't *die*."

"I'll die. Don't let 'em give me any shots."

The pounding drumbeat of my heart was beginning to dull into distant sound.

"Wayne got sick, didn't he?" I asked.

"When?"

"I don't know. When he was here. He was here and he got sick."

"He didn't get sick. He was a little upset. He loves you, you know."

"He got sick. He was looking at the screws in my head and he got sick."

"Now, Tom, don't you say anything to him about that, he feels bad enough as it is."

"Made me sick too," I said. "Am I in Asheville?"

"Yes."

"How long?" I asked. "How long have I been here?"

"A little over two days."

Two days working on three, I thought bitterly. Soon it'll be two months working on six, and after that three more months with a cane, and after that more exercises and after that and after that and after that. There was always an after that. There was always another maze to run. That was what I had tried to explain to Cory. Jesus Christ! Cory. What incredible timing.

"Did you call Cory?" I asked.

I could see the confusion on her face. "No. You asked me not to."

"When?"

"You asked me twice—you insisted. Once in the emergency room and again on the way up here."

I couldn't remember. But I must have been thinking clearer then than now because I wished she were here.

"Would you like for me to call her now?" Mom asked.

Yes, I'd like for you to call her, I thought. I'd like for her to be here. I'd like not to be in this bed. I'd like not to be paralyzed again. I'd like to be able to put my arms around her and hold her and forget all of this. Only I can't put my arms around her and I can't get out of this bed and I can't forget or pretend or hope that this isn't happening.

And what if I did call her, what could she do? Stand by my bed and look at me with the same pitifully helpless look I'd seen on my mother's face. Why put her through that? If she decided not to give her mother a year—if she called—they could tell her. I wouldn't lie to her. If she didn't call, then she'd have her year. Because it would take me that long to get on my feet again—and then I'd call. I'd call as soon as I was on my feet again.

"No," I said. "No, don't call her."

13

"TOM, you're drifting off again. Try to stay awake," she said. "They want you to try to stay awake."

I frowned at her and blinked away the cobwebs. My neck felt fat and I couldn't swallow.

"Did you call Mr. Wakefield in Knoxville?" I asked.

"No, I didn't. It didn't even occur to me," Mom said.

"Well, you better call him and tell him to get himself another man."

"Maybe he could hold the job open. Six months, maybe?" She smiled.

I looked at her with eyes that were serious and weary. "No. Tell him to find someone else. And, Mom, it won't be six months, not this time.

Before she could voice her disagreement, an unfamiliar voice cut into our conversation.

"How's he feeling?"

"Fine," Mom answered, noting the questioning look from me. "You have a roommate. His name is Mr. Perkins."

"Harley, everybody calls me Harley. Mr. Perkins is my old man's name. Man, I'm glad to see you awake, you had us worried there for a while."

"Mr. Perkins stayed awake all night watching you."

I wondered what he had expected to see. I wasn't breathing deep enough to cause any movement, and there were no other signs of life. One second I could have been alive and the next dead, with no visible difference.

"I got run over by a truck and I thought that was pretty bad until your mother told me what happened to you. I didn't think anybody could live with a broken neck."

"They can't," I said, still trying to blink away the haze.

"What?" Harley asked.

"He said he was very lucky," Mom said with a stern look at me. "A very lucky young man."

"I'll say. Hell, that's the way they used to kill people—hang 'em. That's like setting down in the 'lectric chair and coming away with a burned butt."

"And hemorrhoids down to your knees," I added.

"What?"

"He said it's hard for him to talk loud enough for you to hear him," she said with an unmistakable scowl.

"Well, you get some rest and we'll talk later. You've got to see how they've got me strung up. There's ropes and pulleys and weights everywhere, even got a steel pin through my knee—you can see it just pokin' out. I didn't know they had stuff like this."

My head was beginning to pound again and my neck felt bloated to the point of rupture. "Is my neck swollen?" I asked, trying hard to swallow.

"Yes, a little."

"It feels like I'm being choked, like somebody had me by the throat."

"There's a bandage on your throat; maybe the swelling is pulling against the tape."

"On my throat? Then they went in through the front?"

"Yes, Dr. McKinnon thought it would be safer."

"Progress. They operate on your back by going through your

stomach. Well, at least they didn't have to shave my head this time except where the screws are."

"No, but you're going to play havoc combing your hair," Dad said as he and Wayne came into view.

"Yeah, that might prove interesting."

"How you feel?" Wayne asked.

"Well, if I can hang on for a few more rounds I think I can take him." My tongue kept sticking to my mouth, slurring my words.

"You can take him. Just hang in until you figure out his style, then bust him."

"Why don't you go get some sleep and let us visit with him awhile," Dad told Mom.

Wayne and I talked for a while as Dad sat reading a newspaper. At seventeen, Wayne was as tall as I and his frame would carry more weight once he filled out. As we talked, I noticed that he carefully avoided looking at the halo.

"What kinda rig am I in?" I asked. "I know about the halo, but that's about all I know."

"Well," he said, still not looking at the halo, "you're in a body cast that runs from your hips up over your shoulders. And coming straight up out of the back of the cast are two steel rods that bend at a ninety-degree angle over your head— about a foot above your head. Then there are four long screws running from the rods down to the halo. I guess they can adjust the tension on your neck by tightening those screws. At least that's all Dad and I could figure out."

"Well, it's not as bad as it looks," I told him. "I can't even tell it's there. Really. I don't feel it at all. I guess once you're through the little bit of skin on the top of your head there just aren't any nerves to protest. Anyway, I'd rather wear it than have to look at it."

"I can't feel the pin in my knee either," Harley put in. "It's an ugly-looking bugger, but it don't hurt."

"What happened to you?" Wayne asked.

155

"Well, I'll tell you—and it's probably the dumbest thing you ever heard. I work construction, and one morning I had to take a leak so I stepped behind this truck and cut loose. There was a couple of ant hills there and I got interested in drowning them little sons-of-bitches—I was washing away houses and flooding 'em out right and left, chasing 'em all over the place. I got so interested in that that I didn't notice the truck starting to back up until it had knocked me down and was coming up my leg. It finally came to rest smack-dab on my hip bone and it wouldn't have stopped there if I hadn't ahad a hard-on." He laughed.

Wayne glanced at me and grinned.

"That ain't really true. They said if it had come on up onto my stomach it would have killed me so I made up that part about the hard. Told everybody it stopped that truck cold. I'll tell you something that is true—getting it on was bad enough, but driving it back off was pure hell."

"They drove that truck off of you?" Wayne asked.

"Yep, sure did."

"Why didn't they jack it up or something?"

"Nobody had time. That ol' boy that was driving ain't none too smart, and when he heard me yelling and looked in his mirror he just pulled her into low and drove back the way he'd come."

"Damn." Wayne grimaced.

"Well, I used a whole lot stronger language than that."

"I'll bet you did."

"You know what I was worried about? My tally-whacker. I was hurtin' pretty bad and guys were running up there from everywhere, and I just felt embarrassed laying there with my whong hanging out. It's funny what you think about at a time like that, ain't it?"

When I awoke it was dinnertime. I could hear the sounds of Harley eating and the smell of food made me nauseous. I couldn't remember going to sleep. I must have dropped off while Wayne and Harley were swapping stories, but I couldn't remember.

"Do you think you could eat something?" Mom asked.

"No. What time is it?"

"About six."

"You didn't get much sleep."

"I took a quick nap. How about some Jell-O? You should try to eat something."

"I would like something to drink. My mouth feels like a desert."

"Well, let's see. We've got milk and coffee and water. How about milk?"

"Any juice?"

"No, but I could get some."

"Okay, see if they've got some orange juice."

When she returned I was able to force down half a glass of juice before the stinging in my throat made the effort no longer worthwhile.

"They must put a tube down your throat when they operate."

"They do sometimes."

"It sure did tear up my throat."

"Well, remember, they had to push everything to one side in order to reach your spine."

It was an anterior fusion, I realized. They did go in through the front. That was what McKinnon had wanted to do while I was still in Charlotte. I hadn't realized that until now. Was Dr. Walters wrong? Were he and all his big city colleagues wrong and the little country doctor right? I wondered whether, if I had let him do the fusion four years ago, I would be here now. I'd ask him. I'd have to pick the right time because it would mean he would have to admit that a fellow doctor was dead wrong, and it was damn near impossible to get a doctor to do that.

I kept waiting for the right moment, but it never seemed to come. But by the end of the week I was doing well enough for my family to return home, and the pain was no longer a constant wearing force—now it came in swift devastating attacks that left me weak and sick.

I began to try making a game of it—a contest between me and the gods. I could imagine them looking down and throwing one thunderbolt after another. "Wait until he's almost asleep," one would whisper as he sipped something exotic from a jewel-encrusted golden chalice. "Go ahead, why wait," another would say, flicking a speck off his toga. They wagered in gold, and they were arrogant and pompous and supremely confident of victory.

"Damn," I muttered to myself after a particularly prolonged attack. "Ol' Zeus himself must have gotten into the game that time."

"Who?" Harley asked.

"Zeus."

"What's that?"

"It's not a what, it's a who. Zeus is a god."

"The one the Hindus worship?"

"No, the ancient Greeks."

"I thought you was a Hindu."

"I'm not a Hindu."

"You told that lady from dietary you was a Hindu."

"That's because I don't like tomatoes."

"You told that lady from records that you was a Hindu."

"That was to keep all those jack-leg preachers out of here."

"I thought you really was a Hindu. Man, I'm glad to hear you ain't. I ain't been none too comfortable in here with somebody that worships cows."

"Hindus don't worship cows."

"They don't? What do they worship?"

"How the hell would I know?"

"Well, if you don't know, why the hell did you say you were one?"

158

"Look, Harley. When the woman from records was filling out those forms, she asked me my religion and I knew that no matter what denomination I said, the receptionist would put it beside my name and every preacher that comes in here checks that. They make a list of everybody in here that belongs to the same denomination, and most of them will take anything Protestant or anything that comes close to being Protestant, so I decided to pick something most of them knew nothing about. Now you got to admit there ain't been too many Brahmans in here."

"Too many what?"

"Never mind. Now, when dietary got my records they came up to see if I had any special dietary laws I had to adhere to because I was Hindu. Well, I hate tomatoes so I told them my religion forbids me to eat tomatoes. But she put down that I couldn't eat beef either because Hindus don't eat cows. So I had to make up that part about being a member of an offshoot branch that no longer held the cow sacred."

"They ain't gonna believe that for long. You don't look like no Hindu. I asked my sister and she said most Hindus were Indian and you don't look like no Indian I ever seen."

"I told them I converted in college."

"They'll find out."

"What's to find out? You don't know anything about Hindus. I don't know anything about Hindus. The average man doesn't know anything about Hindus except that they don't eat cows. Now you tell me, do Hindus eat tomatoes?"

"How the hell would I know?"

"Exactly. Nobody knows."

"You reckon Hindus eat squash?"

"I don't know."

"I hate squash. Maybe I'll tell 'em I'm a Hindu and I can't eat no squash."

"Forget it."

"No, I'll tell 'em I've changed over since rooming with you. They'll believe that."

159

"Do you want to come back as a cow?"

"Come back?"

"Yes, come back. Hindus believe that you can come back as a cow after you die. You go around spouting off about being a Hindu and somebody up there might take you serious and send you back as a cow."

He thought about it for a while before saying, "Maybe there's some other religion I could tell 'em. Catholic, maybe."

"You don't look Catholic." I laughed.

"You don't look like no Hindu either."

"Catholics eat squash."

"How you know?"

"Everybody knows that. Catholics eat squash and everybody knows it."

"Shit," said Harley.

I heard the click-clack of a woman's heels against the tile floor of the hall as soon as she stepped off the elevator and I followed the sound as she made her way down the hall. Her gait slowed, then picked up again, and I knew she was reading the room numbers above the doors. My heart raced when she paused outside my room and almost stopped beating when she walked past. I listened until the only sound left was the beating of my heart.

I don't know why I kept expecting her to come. She didn't even know I was here, and I wouldn't want her to see me like this anyway. I guess I kept hoping she'd tell her mother no deal and make that call, then she'd know and she'd come. I would have won and what could I do about it? And what could she do about me being here except cry and ask why I didn't let her know. No, it would be best if she didn't come. I wouldn't want her to see me like this. But the next time the elevator stopped and a woman's heels sounded her arrival, I would listen until she passed my door, and each time I would die a little.

"Who you expecting?" Harley asked.

"Nobody."

"Who's Cory?"

"How do you know about Cory?"

"How do I know about her? Man, that's all we heard for the first two days you were here. You 'bout drove me crazy."

"There ought to be some kind of rule about the type of shoes women are allowed to wear in hospitals. They ought to make them go barefoot or wear crepe-soled shoes or something. You can hear them as soon as they hit the floor."

My mood darkened and I didn't feel like talking anymore. That night I woke Harley and asked him to ring for a nurse. I was hot and having trouble breathing. My breath made a rattling, rasping sound in my throat. Dr. McKinnon's diagnosis was arrived at quickly—pneumonia. By the next afternoon, my condition was considered critical and my family was summoned.

When they arrived, my arms and legs were wrapped in towels that had been soaked in alcohol and ice water in an attempt to retard a dangerously high temperature. They did not try to talk to me. They simply told me they were there and would remain at my side. They had learned from past experience that any communication with me at times like this was futile. I had not slept since asking for the nurse. My concentration was directed inward, devoted to kindling the small spark of life remaining in me.

As time passed I grew less able to concentrate, I kept drifting and catching myself just before lapsing into sleep. But I couldn't sleep—I must stay awake.

I heard Dad send Mom to their room and promise to call if there was any change.

I kept drifting and floating and stopping it at the last moment until I was too tired to go on. I tried to blink away the sleep but it wouldn't yield. I opened my eyes wide and blinked hard but the room was dark except for a dim glow somewhere beside and below me. I heard the rustle of paper and I knew Dad was sitting there reading a newspaper.

You better call Mom and tell her, I thought of saying, but

161

why do that, why have her here to see it end?

"Dad," I said, the words rattled out of me like rusty cans. "I'm not going to make it. I'm too tired."

I heard the paper being lowered and I knew he was looking at me.

"You'll make it," he said, and his voice carried no emotion, no alarm.

"Not this time," I told him.

"You'll make it," he said, and I waited for him to come into view but instead I heard the paper again—he was reading! Maybe he didn't believe me. Maybe he didn't realize I meant it and that I was dying. But even if he didn't believe it, he had to know I believed it. He had to know that, and what did he do? What he had always done—he hid. The situation required emotion and he hid. And he said, "You'll make it." What a lousy thing to say. I was dying. I couldn't hold on any longer. I had given up and wanted to use the last of my energy to say farewell to my father and all I got was—you'll make it. A father should have more to say to a dying son. There should be emotion and drama, speeches and tears. There should be confession and forgiveness. Encouragement should be shouted. Hopes should be voiced. Death should be damned, unrealized dreams lamented. A son was dying. This was the time for life—all the grand, sad, beautiful, noble emotions should be stripped raw. Never should two men be closer. You'll make it! What a pitiful thing to say. Well, by God, I would make it. I wasn't about to die like this. Not with somebody sitting in a dark room telling me I was gonna make it. I wasn't going to die!

Pain flicked out in fiery tongues running down my neck and shoulders. I turned my attention and anger toward it, almost welcomed it.

"Tom," I heard her say, and I opened my eyes and saw my mother and it was day again. "Let go, son. You haven't slept in two days. You can't go on like this. You've got to sleep. For God's sake, just let go."

"I can't," I said. "I'm too tired. I can feel it slipping. I can feel my energy seeping out every pore and it's almost gone. I'm beyond sleep. If I let go now I'll sink too deep. It's not sleep that's waiting for me."

She was saying something but I couldn't hear her. I could feel it coming. "Mom, quick, look at the sky. What color is the sky?"

"It's raining," a voice said. Harley probably.

She stood there looking at me and her eyes filled with tears. "It's raining, son."

"I don't care about that. I don't care what it's doing. Just look. See if there's any blue up there—any blue at all. Hurry!"

She stepped away from the bed and I heard her voice far off, like sounds that ride the wind. And then there was nothing.

When I opened my eyes Mom anticipated the question and looked at her watch. "It's six o'clock in the morning and you've been out since ten o'clock yesterday morning."

Before I could ask anything, Dr. McKinnon stepped into view. By the look of him he had been there all night. He slipped a hand beneath my neck and gently pressed.

"I think the worst is over. You just had a little fluid."

"Huh?"

"There was fluid collecting in a pocket between two layers of skin, and it was putting pressure on the cord, making it difficult for you to breathe. That, coupled with pneumonia . . ."

He let the sentence drop and turned to my mother. "Would you excuse us a moment, please."

When she had left the room he said, "When you were in Charlotte, what were you told about a second fusion?"

I looked at him for a moment and wondered how to tell him that I had taken Dr. Walters' advice over his.

This wasn't the right time. I couldn't half think or see and everything he said had an echo. I wanted to be sharp for this— to feel him out carefully. He had taken me by surprise and I

163

wasn't ready for it. Hell, waking up took me by surprise. I thought I was dying.

"I was told . . . that . . . that you wanted to do it but Dr. Walters and some others didn't." My tongue kept sticking to my mouth again, and my head felt like there was something in there expanding.

"What exactly were you told," he insisted, and his tone was sharper than usual.

I tried to remember exactly how Dr. Walters had put it. "I was told that you felt that my neck needed more support and that you wanted to do another fusion. But Dr. Walters and some other doctors thought my neck was strong enough and that I could have a second fusion later if it was necessary, and that any change in the fusion—any weakness—would show up on X-ray. I've gone in for an X-ray every six months since then."

"You were told—" He stopped himself and took in a slow, deep breath. "Weren't you advised that regardless of how the fusion appeared on X-ray, it wasn't solid enough to withstand a blow to the head?"

"No. I was told that it was strong enough, and all we had to watch for were changes."

Something flashed in the depths of his eyes and small ripples ran down the muscle of his jaw. It was the only time I had seen his emotions betray him. Then it was gone.

"Then no one insisted that the fusion was necessary?"

"No," I told him, and things began to blur out of focus.

"All right, you get some sleep and I'll stop back later," he said, and he stepped out of my range of vision.

Well, there it was. He hadn't said it—he hadn't come right out and said it, but Walters was wrong. But more than that— he hadn't presented McKinnon's case the way it should have been presented. He hadn't even presented the facts. If he had, I wouldn't be here now. If he had, I'd be in Knoxville. He had a right to disagree, but he had no right to do this—to keep the facts from me. I could forgive him for being wrong. I could forgive him for making a mistake. But I could not— would not—forgive him this.

I could feel the sleep coming, and I didn't fight it. I felt sick to my stomach, and I didn't want to think about Walters anymore. How could he play with human life? How could he be so sure he was right that he bet my life on it? I felt the anger beginning to grow and I didn't want it now. There wasn't anything I could do about it now. I only wanted to stop feeling, to stop thinking.

I closed my eyes and waited.

14

I STRAINED to hear. I could make out a door being closed, the sound of footsteps, and finally silence. I held my breath so that I could hear better, and then the piercing scream of a woman shattered the silence. The music built to a crescendo and I knew credits were flashing on the screen.

"What happened?"

"He killed her," Harley said.

"Killed who?"

"The blonde. He killed the blonde."

"Dammit, Harley, I don't know which one was blond. I can't see the damn thing. Which one was blond?"

"The one married to the sailor."

"Brenda?"

"Yeah, I guess."

"Who killed her?"

"The guy that walked with a limp."

"Goddammit, Harley! That's it! Television was meant to be seen, not listened to. I never know what the hell's going on."

"Well, I don't know his name."

"You're getting earplugs. Call your sister! Tell her to bring the earplugs."

166

"I thought you enjoyed TV."

"I don't. And I'll tell you something else I don't enjoy. Saturdays. I hate Saturdays. You know why I hate Saturdays? I hate Saturdays because of country western music. I hate that music."

"I thought you liked music."

"I do like music. I even like good country western, but those yokels they have on every Saturday from noon to seven o'clock can't be classified as anything but bad news. They're a disgrace, and they're driving me crazy. Call your sister!"

"Okay. Okay, I'll call her. Why didn't you say something before?"

"I did. I kept asking you to turn it down, change the station, read me the paper—anything. But you never got the message, and who walked with a limp?"

"I don't remember his name, I'm telling you. You really want me to call my sister?"

"Call her! How can you watch a movie for two hours and not know the murderer's name?"

"I didn't know he was the murderer until the end."

"I didn't hear any limp when he crossed the room."

"When?"

"When he killed her!"

"That's right!" Harley exclaimed. "He wasn't limping. The son-of-a-bitch was faking all along."

"Why would he fake it—that doesn't make sense. Are you sure he's the one that did it?"

"Well, it was kinda dark and—"

"Jesus."

I decided to ignore Harley. I felt for the rubber ball I kept by my side and began squeezing it—working the muscles of my right hand and forearm. The strength and range of my right arm had increased at a maddeningly slow pace during the past six weeks. Although there had been a complete return of sensation to all parts of my body, the only muscle response had been in my right arm. The limited movement of my leg stubbornly refused to respond.

167

I had been pleased to find that Curtis Rhinehardt had been replaced by Mrs. Broughton—a fat, jovial woman in her late fifties. But just as her patient effort with passive exercises had not slowed the rapid weight loss, neither had her robust good humor been able to stave off the waves of depression that filled me with doubts as to whether I would ever walk again.

Unlike before, when I had been convinced that, once punctured, the solid wall of paralysis would shatter and fall away, I was denied a single objective toward which to direct my total energy. There was no solid barrier to be punctured. If I concentrated my efforts on strengthening my arm, I felt remiss toward my legs. If, on the other hand, I worked on my legs, their lack of response was frustrating and I feared losing what I had already gained in my arm. I did not have the energy to make a satisfying effort in both areas.

But now I had an idea—a new approach—something I hadn't tried before, and I began thinking about it, trying to bring all my concentration to it, ignoring Harley's attempts at conversation; at first it required effort, but by the second day, if he said anything, I no longer heard him. I could hold the thought as I ate and even during therapy sessions with Mrs. Broughton. I held it until nothing else existed for me. Then it was time to use it. It was time to move my lifeless left leg. My right hand balled into a fist, I bit down hard and tried to bend my knee. Nothing. I tried again and again, until I slumped back in exhaustion.

"Shit," I mumbled.

"What?" Harley asked.

"Nothing," I snorted resentfully.

"What you mad at me for?"

"I'm not mad at you. I'm tired, that's all. I'm tired and I'm out of ideas and nothing works and I quit. I've had it, Harley. I quit."

"You just gonna lay there? You ain't gonna try no more?"

"That's about the size of it."

168

"Aw, you're just saying that because you've been down in the dumps the last couple of days."

"I ain't been down in the dumps. You know what I've been doing? Positive thinking. Mind over matter. And I'll tell you something, Harley—it don't work."

"Huh?"

"I've been thinking, Harley. Just thinking. But I've been doing it for three days. For three days I've been telling myself the leg would move the next time I tried it. I haven't thought about anything else. I saturated my subconscious with the idea. I've seen it move in my mind a thousand times. I've felt it move. Last night I even dreamed it moved. Today I was ready. Ready to try it. No, not try it—do it. Today I was gonna move that leg, and you know what happened, Harley? Nothing! Not one damn thing. I'm tired. I quit. I played my ace and I lost, so I'm hanging it up."

"You won't quit. You'll come up with something."

I refused therapy for the first time that afternoon and tried to accustom myself to doing nothing. It was not the simple task I thought it would be. It took conscious effort to free my mind of the burden of intimidating and harassing a stubborn body into movement. I caught myself thinking that perhaps if I tried just once more, if I put all I had into one final effort—but I had tried. I had put all I could into it, and I had made my final effort. There weren't going to be any more attempts. What more could I do? I had tried to saturate every cell of my body with one simple thought—the leg would move. It didn't move. I hadn't gotten mad. It was a calm, cool approach, not some helter-skelter assault launched in the heat of anger. And maybe that was where I had made my mistake. Maybe if I got mad enough—an insane rage . . . I had tried that, too. I had so alarmed Harley that he called the nurse. That hadn't worked either.

I just had to realize that this was it for me. This was what life was going to be, for as long as it lasted. It should last somewhere around seven years, and I could spend it one of two ways—breaking my back trying to do the impossible, or relaxing and trying to enjoy what was left. They could rig up a television so that I could see it, and if they tried there should be some way to fix something that would allow me to read, I thought, as I studied the familiar chalk-white ceiling. My eyes found a crack that formed a small triangle in the far corner, and I made a mental note not to forget that crack when I built the room.

That ceiling was all I had seen of the room. I had spent weeks—months—staring at it, and it looked as though the smooth, flat plaster would be the easiest surface in the world to walk on. I had gone through the motions of walking a thousand times. I had felt the muscles respond, seen my legs moving forward, heard my feet coming down solid beneath me, and it was always on a surface of smooth, white plaster. I had sworn to build an exact replica of this hospital room one day. To build it upside down and walk on that flawless white ceiling. It would have a gray light fixture in its center and a crack in one corner forming a triangle.

Cory would think I was crazy if I suggested putting a room like that in our home, I thought. But then there wasn't going to be a Cory, or a home, or a room. There wasn't going to be anything but seven years of watching television and reading books and listening to country western music on Saturdays. There wouldn't even be that. Harley wasn't going to be here for seven years. And neither would I. I would be in a home somewhere getting bedsores like Bo. In a home full of old people belching and farting and calling me Sonny. I had almost gotten sick the time we went to see Cory's uncle in one of those places. It reeked of vomit, and human waste, and age. Seven years! I'd be sick for seven years.

"I thought you weren't gonna try no more," Harley said when he noticed my hand rhythmically massaging the red rubber ball.

170

"I tried not trying. It doesn't work either. It's almost impossible to do nothing. It's like trying not to think."

"You got a plan then, right?"

"Right."

"I knew it," Harley said proudly. "I knew you'd come up with something. What is it? What you gonna try now?"

"Faith. Just plain old simple faith, Harley. I'm going to try believing. No matter what anybody says and no matter what happens, I'm going to believe I can beat it. I'm not going to think about it or worry about it or set three-day limits on it. I never had any doubts the first time, and that's where I've been making my mistake. I've been willing to compromise. I've been thinking that *maybe* I could do it again, and if I couldn't then *maybe* I could get along just fine with one arm and both legs or both arms and one leg. Well, that won't get it, Harley. All that'll get you is a bed in some smelly home. No more maybes. No, sir. No more maybes. I'm going to beat it and I'm going to beat it all the way down the line."

In the weeks that followed, I waged a steady, constant campaign against a rebellious body. There were still periods of despondence born of frustration and fatigue, but the dark moods were no longer accompanied by the debilitating self-doubt that had characterized them earlier.

Mom was arranging some flowers she had brought from home. Harley was arguing with his sister over which channel to watch.

"Do you remember the Easter lily you bought me?" Mom asked, stepping back and appraising the arrangement. "You were eight years old then."

"Yep."

"I'll never forget the way you looked carrying it up the front steps. It was bigger than you were. You were having such a tough time with it. You were covered with sweat, and your poor little arms were trembling."

"I carried the blessed thing all the way from town."

"Why didn't you take a cab?" She giggled.

"I didn't have any money. I lacked twenty cents having enough to pay for the monster. I had to act like I was going to cry or the guy wouldn't have sold it to me."

"You didn't!"

"I did. I stuck out my lower lip and started blinking my eyes and said, 'My momma ain't gonna have no flower for Easter,' and some fat lady said, 'Give the kid the flower,' so he did."

She just looked at me and shook her head.

"I didn't realize that thing was as heavy as it was, and about halfway home I decided a card would have done just as well."

"No, it wouldn't," she said. "That's one of my favorite memories."

"Look! Quick, look at that," Harley yelled at his sister, pointing to a pajama-clad man towing a portable IV rod with a bottle swaying from it. "Damn! It's full. Damn the luck."

"What's full, Harley?" his sister asked.

"The bottle. The bottle's full. Do you know what's wrong with that guy? Huh? You got any idea what's wrong with him? Well, I'll tell you what's wrong with him. He's got a strange disease. A *real* strange disease. He has to have that stuff in the bottle to keep going. If it ever runs out, the son-of-a-bitch will stop dead in his tracks. Just like when a car runs out of gas."

"Oh, Harley," she said, making a face.

"It's the God's truth, I swear."

Mom looked down at me knowingly and said softly, "Now, why did you tell him that?"

"Now, what makes you think I told him?"

"I know you."

"Do you think I'd lie to Harley?" I asked in all innocence.

"Yes."

"You're right, I would. But I didn't. It just so happens he got that from the guy's nurse."

"Tom."

"It's the truth if I ever told it. The guy was a missionary to someplace. Albania. He was a missionary to Albania, and while ministering to the sick and misbegotten, he contracted this exotic disease that prevents the body from converting food to energy. So they had to straight-wire him. They have to get his food and energy supply to him by going directly into a vein."

"Tom."

"It's the truth. If I was going to make up a story, I'd sure come up with something more believable than this. Just think about it. The body converts food to energy just like a car converts gas."

"Yes, and if there's no food then the body starts burning its own fat. It doesn't stop like a car. It's called starving."

"Right! You're right, except his body won't burn stored fat. It won't convert food or fat—so what do you get? A person with no energy—*none*—absolutely zero. No energy, no movement. It's crazy, but it's true."

She thought about it and studied my face for any hint of a smile.

"Now, don't you feel bad accusing me of something I didn't do?" I said.

"He wouldn't just stop," she argued. "If it was true, and I'm not saying for one minute that it is, he wouldn't just stop. He would grow tired and then more so and more so as his energy was expended."

"That's probably true. Harley more than likely got the story wrong or just embellished it a little. But either way, I'm not responsible. I had no part of it."

"I don't know," Harley snapped at his sister. "It's got something to do with food and energy. Get Tom to explain it. He's the one that talked to the guy's nurse."

Mom scowled at me as she slowly picked up a towel and dropped it on my face.

"So I lied." I smiled as I pulled the towel off my face.

"You're awful."

"I'm awful? Harley's awful. He's the one who keeps hoping the poor guy'll run out of gas." I laughed. "He watches every move the man makes. It gives him something to look forward to. One day he was way down so I made up a little story to give him something to occupy his mind. You should have heard the whole story; there were Albanian gypsies, lepers, a blond prostitute and—"

"Never mind." She laughed.

Dr. McKinnon cut away the cast and explained that in order for me to be admitted to the rehabilitation hospital it would be necessary that I be under the care of a local doctor. The only doctor he knew in Charlotte was Walters.

"I don't anticipate any problems. The fusion seems solid enough, but I've made arrangements to stay in contact with the hospital, and you know enough to tell if there is any dramatic change. If so, you're to have me notified," Dr. McKinnon said as he steadied my head with one hand and reached for a screwdriver with the other. The chrome screw refused to give and I tensed as my head moved beneath Dr. McKinnon's grip. It was the first time my head had moved since the fall.

"Are you sure you're turning it the right way?" I asked with a nervous laugh. I wanted to alert him to the possibility that he might not be.

"I think so—counterclockwise—I think that's right. I never was very mechanically inclined."

"I wouldn't want you turning it the wrong way and suddenly breaking through and poking me in the brain."

"I don't think there's any chance of that happening." He laughed. It was the first time I had ever heard him laugh. "This should do it," he said, picking up a larger screwdriver.

The screw gave under the fresh assault and I flinched at the slight prick of pain as it wound its way out of my scalp. The remaining screws were less stubborn.

174

"I don't guess there's any need for me to go into my 'Accept-what-you-have-and-learn-to-use-it' speech, is there?" he asked, dabbing at the blood with a gauze pad.

"I don't think so."

"My heart wouldn't be in it anyway—not after the way you proved me wrong the first time. You'll be leaving for Charlotte the day after tomorrow, and about all I can tell you is—how did you phrase it?—take your best shot?"

"I think I did say something like that once."

"Well, you take your best shot and let me hear from you."

"I will."

He looked at me for a moment and his eyes softened as he reached out and squeezed my arm. "Good luck, son."

15

THE ambulance attendants had transferred me from the stretcher to the bed and were making their way out of the room. Mom was looking for a place to put the suitcase and trying to answer the admitting clerk's questions when Don Stirewalt came into the room. He stepped around the stretcher, nodded to Mom, and stared down at me while I continued trying to unfasten the leather straps of my brace.

"Well, what the hell did you do this time?"

I looked up without expression and said, "I fell."

"I know, that's what it says in the chart, but you're talking to me now, and I say it would take more than a simple fall. It's been four years, the graft would have been strong enough to take a fall. It had to be more than that."

"Is that right?"

"Yeah, that's right."

"Hey, Mom," I said. She was still holding the suitcase and pointing to something on the clerk's clipboard. "Don't bother unpacking the bags, the whole thing's been a misunderstanding. I sure am glad you came by," I told Stirewalt. "I might have lain around here for God knows how long thinking I was paralyzed."

176

Stirewalt stopped the smile that tugged at the corners of his mouth. "You want to quit playing smartass and tell me how you managed to screw up all the work I put in on you?"

"I fell."

"I see. You simply fell down, and that's it?"

"I didn't say there was anything simple about it. But then, there wasn't anything spectacular about it either. I guess it was just your average run-of-the-mill, everyday fall-down-the-steps-hit-your-head-on-the-bumper-of-the-car type fall."

"Still the same ol' hard nose, aren't you?" he said with a broad grin. "Why didn't you say that to start with?"

"Why didn't you help me with this brace instead of standing there asking silly questions?"

"Oh, I couldn't do that," he said with mock gravity. "You see, you're here to become self-sufficient, and the only way you're going to accomplish that is to learn to do things for yourself. I couldn't help you with that brace. Oh no, uh-uh."

"You haven't changed a whole hell of a lot yourself," I said, and studied his face to see if he was serious. "I think I used the wrong word. Help's not what I meant. Teach is the word I meant to use. You need to *teach* me to get out of this thing," I said with mock formality. "You see, this is the first time I've had it on and, even though I've only got one hand that's working, I'm sure I could manage to get out of this thing once somebody shows me how."

"Well, now that you put it that way." He laughed and began unbuckling the brace.

"Methodist," I heard Mom tell the clerk as Stirewalt placed the brace on the bedside cabinet.

"I'll give her all that information later," I told Mom.

"Well, let's see just what we've got to work with," Stirewalt said, holding out a huge hand. "Squeeze."

"Wait a minute," I told him. "Mom, I'll take care of that, just let it go for now."

"I don't mind. You go ahead with Mr. Stirewalt."

"Squeeze," Stirewalt repeated.

I glared at him. "You couldn't wait, could you? Now you see what you've done?"

"What?" he asked, glancing uneasily around the room.

"Now, thanks to you, I've got to eat tomatoes."

He turned slowly and looked at me with probing distrust. "There's nothing on earth worse than stewed tomatoes."

"You know, sometimes you don't make a damn bit of sense."

"Gimme that hand," I said.

I knew I didn't have the strength to apply as much pressure as would be needed, so I grabbed the middle fingers of Stirewalt's outstretched hand and began to squeeze. I could feel Stirewalt's wedding ring beneath my grip and saw him stiffen.

"That's enough," he said.

I stared at him, a big grin on my face, and increased the pressure.

"Okay! Okay!" he said, coming up on his toes and prying my fingers open with his free hand. He stood there rubbing his hand for a minute. "That was a mistake," he said, breaking into a broad smile. "Now let's check those hamstrings."

He moved to the foot of the bed and picked up my leg. As he locked the knee and began to lift the leg, he glanced quickly at me and I watched him without expression. The leg came up easily. The hamstrings offered no protest and it surprised him. I continued to show no expression as Stirewalt brought the leg up to its limit.

"That's as far as it'll go," I snapped. "I ain't no ballerina."

"Somebody's done a damn good job on you," he said, lowering my leg.

"I had a therapist this time instead of that little fag."

"Well, they sure kept you loose. How 'bout the shoulders?" he asked as he moved up the bed and reached for my arm.

"Let's wait until tomorrow," I told him. "I'm tired, it's been a long day."

"Okay. Sure. It must have been a long trip for you. Get some rest and I'll see you in the gym tomorrow."

The following day Stirewalt's slow, probing examination revealed that although there had been a complete return of sensation, motor response was limited to my right arm and to patches of muscle in my right leg.

That evening one of Dr. Walters' associates did a complete physical on me. I was glad Walters had sent him instead of coming himself. There was nothing I could say to Walters that would get him to admit to more than an error in judgment. He would never admit to misrepresenting the facts, and even if he did, it wouldn't change anything.

Still, I would like to see him. To see if there was anything in his eyes or his face that would reflect guilt, or if there was something there I missed the first time—something that should have alerted me to the flaw in him that allowed him to hold his specialty so superior to another that he gambled human life on it.

We began a program that allowed me to set my own pace and employed every therapeutic device at Stirewalt's command. In the mornings I was wheeled to the gym on a stretcher and transferred to a wheelchair for the afternoon session. Stirewalt scheduled me for twice-a-day sessions of physical therapy, hydrotherapy, and heat treatments.

The old rivalry between us was still there, but it became evident during the first few weeks that I did not have the energy to bring to it I once had had. I was exhausted most of the time and complained to Stirewalt that a night's sleep did nothing to replenish me. I woke up exhausted. It was not unusual for Stirewalt to leave me on the mats with instructions to continue a particular exercise, only to return and find me asleep. This angered me more than it did Stirewalt, and when he suggested shortening the sessions I bitterly refused.

To get me out of the gym and afford me a chance to rest, he began taking me with him to the staff lounge on coffee breaks. Administration voiced some disapproval, but he ignored them just as he had in the past.

We were in the staff lounge when I looked up with surprise

to see Rick standing in the door. The last time we had seen each other was a couple of weeks before graduation when we had pitched a monumental drunk because of Rick's impending departure for the air force.

"Well, it's about time you showed up. Where the hell have you been?"

"You know where I've been. Officers' training school. Why the hell didn't you write?"

I rolled my eyes toward the ceiling. He knew I hadn't been able to write. "I suppose you're an officer now?" I said.

"An officer *and* a gentleman."

"God help us."

"I'll thank you to keep a civil tongue in your head and keep in mind who you're addressing. Son, you happen to be in the presence of America's new deterrent. The air force's answer to the yellow peril, the Communist horde, and creeping moral decay. I'm the ultimate weapon. I am the answer."

"To what?"

"Who knows?" He shrugged. "I'm trained for anything. They even taught me to dance."

"Well, dance on over here and meet Don Stirewalt. You've heard me speak of Rick Tucker," I said to Stirewalt. "Well, that's it."

Rick and Stirewalt shook hands and they talked about military service for a while before Rick said to me, "You're not going to believe which school they're sending me to—fuel supply. Do you believe that?"

"You're kidding. You've gotta be kidding."

"I swear." He laughed.

"We're in trouble," I told Stirewalt. "We're in serious trouble."

"Fuel supply, now, not development—*supply,*" Rick added.

"I don't care, we're still in trouble. Ain't that just like the military!"

"You want to let me in on the joke?" Stirewalt said.

Rick and I looked at each other and grinned.

"You tell him," Rick said.

"Okay. We must have been sixteen or seventeen at the time. I was building this rocket and I put the genius here in charge of developing the fuel because his father ran a drugstore and that gave him access to all kinds of chemicals. So, with all that to choose from, what does he come up with? A mixture of sulfur, charcoal, and saltpeter, which is nothing less than plain old gunpowder."

"You said your valve could handle it," Rick put in. Then to Stirewalt he added, "He had me convinced that that damn valve of his was gonna revolutionize rocketry. We were gonna have the first solid fuel rocket—get our pictures on the cover of *Time*, win scholarships to MIT—and I believed him."

"What happened?" Stirewalt asked.

"What didn't happen," Rick said. "Go on, Einstein, tell the man."

"We've got this friend—Jimmy Casteen—who lived on a farm just out of town, so I asked him—"

"Conned him," Rick corrected. "You conned him."

"Okay, so I lied a little."

"You've got to understand that Jimmy Casteen's afraid of everything," Rick explained to Stirewalt. "But most of all, he's afraid of Tom."

"Usually when we got together Jimmy came out on the short end of the stick—it wasn't planned that way, it just happened. So, anyway, he agreed to let us fire the rocket on his father's farm and everything was going fine. We set it up in a field and got down in a drainage ditch. You should have seen it—six feet tall, four inches in diameter, standing there with the sun gleaming off it—it was something to see. Rick was so moved by the sight of it that he wouldn't let me fire it until he made a speech about the future of mankind, pioneers, and new frontiers."

Rick shrugged. "I got carried away. I got caught up in the spirit of it all."

"Well, when I finally threw the switch, nothing happened.

It just shuddered and fell over on its side. It was pointed straight at us and we were afraid to get out of the ditch. Standing up, it was beautiful—lying down, it was a six-foot stick of dynamite. About the time we decided it would be safe to go see what was wrong, it started trembling and shaking and inching its way toward us. It started skipping and hopping across the ground, and old Jimmy bolted straight upright and just stood there moaning. He wasn't moving above the ankles and he wasn't headed anywhere, but his feet were patting the ground to beat hell. Then it started to roar, and Jimmy pissed all over himself and fainted dead away just as she blew.

"We brought Jimmy around and raised up out of that ditch— you should have seen it—"

"There was a hole out there you could drop a car in," Rick added. "Then Jimmy looked over in the other field and mumbled 'Oh, my God' and fainted again."

"That scared me," I admitted. "I mean that scared the hell out of me. I looked over there and the tractor Jimmy's old man had been on was moving right along, only Jimmy's old man wasn't on it anymore."

"I thought we'd killed him."

"I did too. We blew him right out of the saddle—knocked him out cold."

"We didn't know what to do. Jimmy was passed out, his old man was knocked out—dead, for all we knew—and the field was on fire."

"Plus every window was blown out of the house and there were dead chickens everywhere. And in the middle of all that, Rick turns to me and says, 'Does this mean we don't get our pictures on the cover of *Time?*' "

"And Tom looked at me just as serious and said, 'Not necessarily.' "

"We had to pay for all that, and Jimmy wasn't allowed to run around with us for a while."

"And I wasn't allowed in the drugstore anymore," Rick said.

182

Later, when Stirewalt excused himself, Rick pushed me back to my room and I sat in the wheelchair listening to him talk about his experiences in basic training. There was a lull in the conversation, and he found something interesting about a button on his cuff and toyed with it.

"I was sorry to hear about you and Cory," he finally said. "What happened?"

"Cory's mother. She wanted us to wait a year, and I wasn't willing to wait. I might have been, if it had been legitimate, but it wasn't. It was just a stall, and I backed off from her a hundred times. I just got tired of backing away."

"Have you heard from her?"

"No. At first I thought I might have, but then . . ." I let it drop and wedged a finger beneath my chin and pulled down on the chin cup of the brace. "Her pride was hurt and she's not sure exactly what she owes her mother."

"Why don't you call her?"

"And say what? Come watch me put myself back together? No, thanks. The days are long enough as it is. I don't think I could take it if she was here waiting."

"So, where do you go from here?"

"I don't have any choice. First I get this body of mine in working order, then I call Cory, and then I find a job. I'll put it all together again, but I've got to do it one step at a time." I reached down, picked up my limp left arm, and repositioned it in my lap.

"How long do you think you'll be here?"

The implication of the question was clear. Cory might not be waiting. She could be having an active social life already, and there was no assurance that she would be there when I did call.

"I don't know," I confessed. "It's slow but it'll come."

She would be there, I told myself after Rick had gone. I did not allow myself to think about her very often but, sitting alone in the empty, quiet room, I thought of her—the music

183

in her laughter, the way she moved, the smell of her hair, the way her eyes became smoky after lovemaking. The urge to call her was strong. I looked at the bedside table to see if there was any change for the phone. There wasn't. I'd have to look in the drawer, and as I moved my left arm so that I could reach the wheel of the chair, I sat looking at it. And then at my legs.

I felt my mood darken. I didn't want her to see me this way. I reached for the call buzzer and mashed the plunger. She would be there, I told myself. I'd call her as soon as I was on my feet again. In the meantime I simply had to believe she'd be there. Nothing could be gained by thinking otherwise, and nothing would be lost by believing. I believed I would walk again, and I would. I believed she'd be there, and she would.

"Yes," the nurse said.

"Take me to the gym."

16

USING the brush like a spoon, I dipped it deep into the can, bringing out as much of the thick green paint as I could. I held it above the place where the two small boards failed to meet and let the paint slide down the brush into the slender opening. It filled the ridge where the boards joined, spread into the opening, and filled it. The structure was solid for a moment; then a small bubble appeared in the fragile web of paint and began to grow and spread until the web collapsed, dripping slender green fingers into the narrow gap.

I dropped the brush to one side and slumped back in the chair.

"You're late," Stirewalt said, stepping into the room.

"I wanted to finish this," I said without turning around.

Stirewalt walked over and looked with distaste at the awkward green structure on the workbench.

"What is it?" he inquired slowly, looking over his glasses at me. His mouth curled as though he had encountered a repugnant odor.

"Whadda ya mean, what is it?" I snapped.

"I mean, what the hell is it supposed to be?"

"You mean to stand there and tell me you don't know what that is?"

He moved around to the other side and studied it thoughtfully, then he cut his eyes at me and shook his head.

"Nope. I wouldn't even guess."

"It happens to be a birdhouse," I explained indignantly.

He stared at me, a big grin on his face. "You're kidding. That's what you've been working on all these weeks?"

"That's it," I said proudly.

"None of the pieces fit."

I shrugged.

"One side of the roof—I guess it's the roof—reaches the floor and the other side barely reaches the wall."

I nodded with a conciliating smile.

"There's no door," he cried with a twinge of alarm.

"So?"

"So, you're supposed to bore a hole in the front."

"You ever try to use a brace and bit with one hand?"

"I guess not," he conceded.

"Ever try to drive a nail with one hand?" I asked. "I had to glue all that together."

"Well, there's a crack in the roof," he said. "Right there where those two pieces are supposed to meet."

"I know there's a crack in the roof," I said indulgently.

"Maybe if you dabbed a little paint . . ." he said, reaching for the paintbrush.

"I've already tried that," I explained. "It'll just run down inside. There's more paint inside the damn thing than there is outside."

"Well, if you'd just cut off that one long piece—"

"Nope. That's it," I insisted. "Do you know how long it takes me to saw through one of those boards? Days. Saw a while— rest a while. No, sir. That's it. You're looking at a finished product. One genuine, handmade birdhouse. And it's probably the most expensive birdhouse you'll ever see. I figured up how much occupational therapy costs per hour and how many hours it took me to finish that thing, and it comes out to better than six hundred dollars."

"Jesus."

"And now I'm finished with it, and I'm finished with occupational therapy. It's a waste of time and energy, and I don't have a lot of either one—not to mention money."

"Mrs. Turnage is going to raise hell if you stop coming."

"Let her. I shouldn't have let you talk me into coming in here anyway."

"I thought we could avoid a run-in with administration."

"I haven't figured out yet why they call this occupational therapy. Building birdhouses is not my occupation," I said, looking at the small wooden house. "If administration raises hell, I'll bring 'em around here and show 'em this and tell 'em they were training me to be a slumlord."

"If you hang that thing you'll be creating a slum all right." He laughed.

I flinched and reached for my left arm. I ran a hand up and down it briskly.

"Your arm bothering you again?" he said with concern.

"Yeah."

"Let's get a little heat on it and see if it'll ease up," he said as he pulled my chair away from the cluttered bench.

A few minutes later I was stretched out on a table watching Stirewalt adjust gauges whose wires led to the soft pads wrapped around my arm and shoulder. I felt the soothing warmth begin to penetrate my aching arm.

"It should start to ease in a minute," he said, seating himself on an adjoining table. He picked up my brace and began toying with the adjustments.

"I've been meaning to ask you for a long time—what ever happened to Bo?" I asked.

"Bo?" Stirewalt asked with a puzzled look.

"Bo Boman."

187

He frowned and shook his head. Then his expression lightened and he said, "Hal. You mean Hal Boman."

"Yeah, I'd forgotten his name was Hal. All I ever called him was Bo."

"He's dead."

"Dead?"

"He left just after you did, and it must have been about a year later that I heard he had died."

"How? What killed him?"

"Pulmonary embolism."

"What's that?"

"A blood clot in the lung."

I started to say I was sorry. It was automatic. It was what you always said when someone died. But I didn't say it.

"I'm glad," I said. "I'm glad it was quick and I'm glad he's out of it. I'm only sorry it took as long as it did. He said that's what would happen. He said one day a blood clot would float up out of his leg and hit something vital."

"It wasn't hard to predict," Stirewalt said quietly.

"Where was he? In a home?"

"Yes."

I tugged at the wrappings on my arm and Stirewalt found something to adjust on my brace. Neither of us spoke for a while.

"How about Glen?" I said finally. "Glen Teeter?"

"I don't know," Stirewalt said without looking up. "I don't know what happened to him. I think they committed his old man."

"Couldn't happen to a more deserving person."

"Why the hell didn't you stay in touch?" he said, glancing up from the brace.

"I did," I argued. "I came by."

"One time, one lousy time."

"Maybe I was afraid to come back after the way you showed your ass."

"What?" he growled. "What the hell are you talking about?"

"You know what I'm talking about. When I walked in the gym, you grabbed me by the hand and yelled, 'Hey, everybody, would you believe this is a quad!' and took off across the room like a bat outta hell."

"So?" He chuckled. "What's wrong with that?"

"Did it ever occur to you that I had just gotten rid of the cane? That I'd never tried to run—didn't even know if I could, and there you were dragging me across the gym. And when you jumped that poor son-of-a-bitch lying on the mat, I almost had a heart attack."

Stirewalt laughed.

"I can still see the look on that guy's face. He was terrified. You might not have known I couldn't run, but he didn't have any questions about it. One look at me coming across that gym like a spastic giraffe, and there wasn't much room for doubt."

Stirewalt's massive frame shook with laughter.

"It's not funny." I chuckled. "And I came one other time— to talk to Allen McDevitt. Why'd you call me anyway? I didn't know what to say to that guy."

"I didn't give a damn what you said to him. I just wanted him to see you walking around."

"Did it work?"

"I don't know. He transferred to a hospital in New York a week or so later; but that reminds me, there's someone here I want you to meet. Cindy Davis."

"Shit. I hate that. I hate it when you ask me to talk to some-body. What the hell am I supposed to say?"

"Who the hell's asking you to say anything? I just said I want you to meet her. If anything, she could give *you* a few words of advice."

"Well, good, there for a minute I thought you were going to say you just wanted her to see me walk."

"Yeah? Well, I would. I really would like for her to see that, but since you don't seem able to manage it since you screwed up all the work I put in on you, I'll settle for—"

"You could show her my birdhouse."

"That damn birdhouse—" He stopped and shook his head. "I don't need to show her anything. That girl's a champion—a real champion."

"What's wrong with her?"

"She's a quad. She was in here a little over a year ago and she's back for a little therapy and to be fitted for new braces."

"She's on leg braces?" I asked with surprise.

"No. Hand splints. She had no return below the shoulders," he said, standing up and turning off the machine.

"What happened to her?"

"Stupid! One of those goddamn stupid kid things. The night of her high-school prom her date—never had a drink in his life—gets shit-faced and smashes up the car. Didn't get a scratch, but Cindy ends up with a broken neck," he said, unwrapping my arm. "Maybe if she'd been drinking . . . maybe . . . but it doesn't work that way, does it?"

"No."

"Well, by God, she's a scrapper, I'll tell you that," he said as he helped me slide off the table into the wheelchair. "She didn't have any more return than Boman—a little shoulder and elbow movement—and she just finished her first year of college."

"You're kidding."

"No, I'm not. I told you, the girl's a champion. We fitted her with hand splints, she learned to write and . . . come on, I want you to meet her," he said, wheeling me out of the room.

I don't know what I expected but, whatever it was, Cindy Davis didn't fit it. She was sitting in a wheelchair; her hands, encased in metal splints, were folded in front of her, resting on a wooden writing board that lay across the arms of the chair. Her hair was midnight black, cut short and curling in around a face that was pale and strained, but shining. Her eyes were sea green, confident, intelligent, and sparkling with life. Her lips were parted in a smile that mixed pleasure at meeting me with compassion for the circumstances of our meeting.

Stirewalt introduced us, and she broke into a broad smile.

"You should charge him for the use of your name," she said. "He uses it frequently."

"Abuses it at times," I said with a smile.

"There were times I hated you, you know. He measured my efforts against yours so often." Her eyes flicked almost unnoticeably to my legs and a shadow crossed her face. She glanced back at my legs and then turned an accusing stare at Stirewalt.

"He did—he could," Stirewalt said suddenly, as if he had been stuck with something sharp. "He could walk. This is the second time for him. Tell her," he said, nodding at me the way you do a child when you want an affirmative answer.

I looked at him as though he was speaking a language I had never heard.

"Well, tell her," he snapped.

"Tell her what?"

"Tell her how you walked."

"You mean before I got hurt?"

"No, I mean after you got hurt."

"After I got hurt I was paralyzed, but I'm getting better."

"You bastard," he said, and I saw Cindy smother a smile.

"I've been in a home for three years, but I've begun to get some return so they brought me back," I explained to Cindy. Then I looked at Stirewalt. "Is that what you meant by second time?"

He exhaled loudly, and Cindy couldn't hold back the grin. She began to giggle.

We talked for a while. Stirewalt explained why I was back, and I confessed to having walked after the first accident. Cindy and I agreed to meet in the dining room for dinner, and then it was time to return to the gym.

I flexed my right arm and winked at Cindy. "I think I just might make twenty-five pounds today."

"I don't think so," Stirewalt said.

"Watch me."

"No way. You'll never do it."

"I'll do it."

"Not twenty-five pounds, not today."

"Cup of coffee says I will."

"You're on," he said.

17

THE white plastic brace lay beside me on the cool gray mat, but I was no longer aware of the mat's coolness. My chest rose and fell with the quick, shallow breaths of exhaustion. My cut-off jeans were stained with sweat. The red sweatshirt, with the sleeves cut off at the elbows and the word STOLEN stenciled across the back, clung to a wet body. I was tired, but I was always tired when I got to the mats. I spent an hour here after each session with Stirewalt. An hour devoted to a total, concentrated effort at moving my left leg. It was a painful, frustrating effort that drained the last vestige of energy from me at the close of each day.

Damn that nurse, I thought, wiping at a trickle of sweat running down my neck into a pool collecting in the hollow of my throat. I shouldn't have lost my temper. I should have played it as I always had. I had done what I had been refusing to do for weeks—I had wasted energy.

The long, slow march of days had stretched into weeks and the weeks into months—months of sweating and straining, months of ignoring pain and fighting fatigue, months filled with endless hours of repetition and failure, frustration and anger, months of agonizing effort that had yielded nothing—nothing until the last few weeks, when my left arm had suddenly sprung to life and was responding to Stirewalt's carefully regimented exercises.

Nurse Jarvis had picked that time to insist that I begin one of her classes—to learn to dress myself with one hand. I had tried repeatedly to explain to her that my energy was extremely limited and that if the orderly continued helping me dress, then I could use that energy to regain the use of my left arm and her class would no longer be necessary. My explanation fell on deaf ears. Nurse Jarvis had been put in charge of the newly initiated classes, and she was seeking recruits. She greeted me each morning undeterred. She was immune to reason, impervious to anger, and incapable of understanding the logic of my argument.

This morning she had forbidden the orderly to assist me and stood there smugly swinging my jeans from her fingertip. I snatched the pants from her, determined to put a stop to her senseless harassment by dressing myself and proving once and for all that I didn't need her damn class. I used my hands to pull my left leg up and, holding it in place with one hand, I lassoed my foot with the jeans. Then I worked my right leg into them and, by pulling them and rocking from side to side, slid them up over my hips.

I pulled and tugged at my left leg until I finally gripped it by the ankle. I held it with my weak left hand and tried to lasso my foot with the small circle of a sock's mouth. I lost my grip, my leg sprang forward, knocking me back on the bed. Nurse Jarvis smiled and walked out of the room.

I was overdue at the gym, and when Stirewalt came looking for me, he found me sprawled awkwardly across the bed—sound asleep, with one leg hanging off the bed and a sock dangling from my foot.

Damn that nurse, I thought again as I slid my right foot into position, flat against the mat. I had hoped to be rid of her. If I could dress myself I wouldn't need the orderly, and Jarvis would have no control over me. But it would be months before I would be able to get socks on unaided, and she would be there every morning.

I wiped the sweat away from my eyes with the back of my hand and readied myself for one last assault on my leg. The muscles of my right leg tensed, forcing the heel deep into the mat as I strained to bend my left knee. My elbows dug into the mat. The muscles of my jaw jittered and danced. I could feel it coming—just a little more effort. The knee was coming off the mat. I poured all my strength into the effort. The muscles of my right leg began to quiver and my foot suddenly lost its bite on the mat and slipped, slamming my leg onto the mat. I brought my right leg back into position and again it slipped. And again. And again. Until the muscles hardened into tight knots and it refused to respond. Frustration swept over me in waves. I lay there breathing deeply through my nose, my lips pressed together so tight that they began to tremble.

"There's no shame in tears," a voice said.

I looked up to see Cindy sitting beside me. I had not heard the gentle whir of the electric motor on her chair. I shook my head.

"I don't believe anybody's ever come through here without leaving a few behind. It's part of a package deal—no extra charge," she said with a sad, gentle smile.

I looked at her sitting there at the end of the mats. I noticed the dark circles under her eyes and pale skin pulled tight across high cheekbones. She was as tired as I was, and I don't know why I was surprised, because she matched me hour for hour in the gym. She must have been beautiful once, I thought. When her face was full, when her body was full.

"I guess so," I said, and my breath came in quick, short puffs. There was still some of the beauty there, in her face, in her eyes. A fire still danced in the depths of her eyes. And

195

I wondered how she did it. For me there was still hope—still the possibility of some return. But for her . . . Maybe that would be the time for tears—when there was no more hope.

I looked at her eyes and the life in them, and there was something beautiful, something noble about her spirit standing tall amid the rags of her flesh. I would have liked to tell her that I was moved by her courage. I wanted to say something about the nobility of her spirit, about bravery and courage and fighting the good fight; but it would embarrass us both, so it would go unsaid.

"I'll tell you something," I said, looking around the gym to see if anyone was listening and leaning closer to take her into my confidence, "I do cry. But the accident left my system all screwed up," I whispered.

She leaned forward and concern was evident in her expression.

"Tears don't come out of my eyes anymore, they come out my pores."

She frowned slightly, thinking.

"I call it sweat."

"Oh, you're hopeless." She laughed. Pressing a lever with the palm of her hand, she backed away from the mats. "They're closing up. I'll see you in the dining room in a few minutes."

I slid off the mats into my chair and rolled down the hall and into the dining room. The two long tables running down the center of the room were already full. I looked around the noisy room and saw her sitting at a small table in the far corner. When I reached the table, an aide set a tray in front of me. Removing the metal hood that covered the meal, I looked down with disgust at a plate containing a large serving of stewed tomatoes.

"The end of a perfect day." I exhaled in exasperation.

"Well, I don't know about that," she said, "but it's the end of my last day here. I'm going home in the morning."

"Really? That's great."

196

"I think it's about time. I was only supposed to be here a couple of weeks but, thanks to kidney stones and infections, it's been almost four months."

"I know you're going to be glad to get out of here," I said, wearily slumping back in my chair.

"I've missed a semester of school, and I think that's what I'm looking forward to most—getting back to school and my friends. And that reminds me, I've been meaning to ask you if you know Brad Brockman. He's from your hometown, and he's been a great help to me on campus. I don't know what I would have done without him."

I shook my head. "I don't think I know any—*Bradley!* Bradley Brockman? Crazy Bradley?"

She giggled at my reaction. "I don't think so. I've never heard him called anything but Brad, and he certainly isn't crazy."

"Big guy? Weighs about two forty, brown curly hair?"

"Yes."

"That's Herb Brockman's little brother. I grew up with Herb."

Well, he isn't little anymore."

"He never was. He's been that big since he was fourteen, and so has his brother."

"Why do you call him Crazy Bradley?"

"Because he is. He was always causing us trouble. Always," I said. "Listen, one night a bunch of us were staying over at Herb's—we were going to get up early to go hunting or something—and we decided to sample some of his old man's liquor. Well, Bradley got bombed—I mean, he wasn't even with us, he just kept hanging around. So we put him to bed, and during the night he started to get up to go to the bathroom but his leg was asleep—we had laid him on it or something. When he stood up his leg just wasn't there, and he fell over a table and broke a lamp and started yelling, 'Polio! Polio!' Now, what in God's name made him think he had polio? There hadn't been a case of polio in that town since before he was born. Woke up the whole damn family. Scared his mother to death. When she got in there, he was sitting on the floor holding his leg, big tears running down his face—still yelling 'Polio! Polio!' "

"I can't believe it's the Brad I know."

"Does he have some kind of breathing problem?" I asked. "Does he have trouble breathing when he gets excited—turns blue sometimes?"

She nodded. "He has trouble breathing sometimes."

"Well, that's Bradley."

"I guess it's the same person." She laughed. "I can't wait to see him again. Crazy Bradley, huh?"

"Yeah," I said, looking at the tomatoes. "I can't eat this. I'm too tired to even try. I think I'll grab a shower and turn in," I told her, pushing myself away from the table. "I'll see you before you leave."

I rolled down the hall and into the bathroom. I snapped off the collar and tossed it in the sink. I would need some help transferring to the waterproof shower chair, so I pushed the call buzzer. I struggled out of my shirt, tossed it in the sink along with the brace, and waited.

The door opened and in walked a huge black orderly, who broke into a broad toothy grin.

"Man, you sho' play hell with my schedule. Why you don't do like everybody else?"

"Maybe I hear a different drummer." I shrugged.

"I sho' wish you'd get in tune with the rest of the band," he said, bending down on one knee and unlacing my shoes. "You ain't scheduled for a bath till eight fifteen."

"I can't stay awake till then. I don't even know if I'll make it through this shower."

He smiled sheepishly at me as he effortlessly lifted me from one chair to the other.

"I hear Jarvis got the best of you this mornin'."

198

"She didn't get the best of me. I just bit off more than I could chew, and I've been paying the price all day."

"You look it. You gonna mess around and let dat woman whup you."

He adjusted the shower, tested it with his hand, and rolled me under the needle-fine jets of refreshing hot water. Sitting down in my wheelchair, he stretched his long legs and lit a cigarette. When he finished, he snuffed it out on the side of the sink.

"Hey, deacon," he shouted above the drumming of the shower, "I been thinkin'."

"Not while you're at work, I hope," I yelled back.

"Aw, man, be serious. I think I know how we can beat ol' Jarvis."

"I'm listening."

"Why don't I get you dressed at night 'fore you goes to bed."

I reached up and cut off the shower.

"Whadda ya think?" he asked eagerly as I rolled out of the steaming stall and reached for a towel.

I looked thoughtfully at him for a moment.

"Won't work."

"Why?" he asked.

"Jarvis wants me to be able to do it myself, and she won't get off my back until I can."

"You ain't strong enough. You done tol' her dat a thousand times."

"No, I'm strong enough. I'm strong enough to get into everything but my socks without using too much energy."

"You still gonna need some help with your socks and shoes."

"No, no, I'm not." I grinned at him. "I'm not gonna wear socks. Hell, I went halfway through college not wearing socks."

"You gots to wear shoes. They won't let you come in the gym without 'em. How you gonna get down there and tie 'em?"

"Simple, my dear Watson, simple. Loafers. I got a pair of

199

loafers in my closet. So tomorrow morning I get up, get dressed—*by myself*—and roll out of there leaving Jarvis with nothing left to sell. She's made my life miserable for the last morning. Now, ol' partner, I think I'll go to bed."

18

BUOYED by water, I supported my weight with my right leg, standing waist deep in the pool. Reassured by my hand beneath her stomach, ten-year-old Althea Biggers let her chubby body float lazily in the warm water.

The slow passing of months had brought a resurgence of energy with which I had painstakingly hammered new strength into the muscles of my arms and shoulders. And now, by assisting Stirewalt with other patients, I could spend more time in the pool, where I hoped to elicit a similar response from my legs.

I lifted Althea high in the water and marveled at the facility with which I did it. Easing her back into the water, I lowered her hips to just beneath the surface and, taking care to let the water absorb the force of the blow, I brought my free hand down across her bottom with a resounding slap.

"Kick!" I ordered above her squeals.

She halfheartedly kicked one leg. I brought my hand up again and held it threateningly above her. Giggling, she began to move both legs.

"You love me, don't you?" she asked, looking over her shoulder.

"Certainly not!" I laughed. "Now come on, *kick!*"

"Yes you do. You say you don't, but you really do."

"How could I possibly love something like you. Look at yourself—you're a mess," I said, picking up a wet curl and letting it fall back on her shoulder.

"I don't know how you do it, but you do."

"What I'd love is to see you walk, and the only way to do that is to kick those legs."

"But it hurts." She pouted.

"I know it hurts, but if you want to walk again you've got to do it."

"No I don't," she said flatly. "I'll walk in heaven and I won't have to kick, either."

"Who told you that?"

"It's true," she said, setting her tiny jaw.

"Where did you hear that?"

"Mrs. Smathers told me."

"And who is Mrs. Smathers?"

"My Sunday school teacher."

"God save us from well-meaning Sunday school teachers," I moaned.

"It's true," she said smugly. "It's in the Bible."

"The Bible, huh? You want to talk about the Bible—I'll tell you about the Bible. Three score and ten, that adds up to seventy, and seventy years is how long the *Bible* says you should live. That leaves you sixty years to go, and that's a long time to wait."

"I don't care," she said stubbornly.

"Well, I do. Now kick."

"No, I won't. It hurts."

"Let me put it to you another way—I'm older than you so I'll probably die before you, which means I'll get to heaven before you, and if I'm watching the pearly gates the day you arrive—*you don't get in!* And the reason you don't get in is because you didn't try hard enough when you were back on earth."

"You won't be watching the gate," she said knowingly. "Saint Peter does that."

"Yes, he does," I conceded. "You're absolutely right. He's the head man, but he's not there all the time—I mean, what kind of heaven would it be if he had to work twenty-four hours a day? He has to have some time to play his harp or whatever it is saints do. And when he's not there, somebody else is, and I just might be that somebody. Now, give me ten good kicks and you can go."

"You really wouldn't let me in?" she asked with a frown.

"Nope."

She looked thoughtfully at me and considered the possibility.

"Just ten and then I can go?"

"Just ten," I told her.

I made her start over twice and then motioned for the lift. I sat her on the stretcher and stepped back as it began to rise from the pool. Althea sat on the edge holding on to one of the chains leading up from the canvas stretcher, her legs dangling over the side.

"I know you love me," she said with a broad grin.

I winked at her and turned my attention back to my own exercises.

Later that day I positioned my chair at the parallel bars and waited for Stirewalt. I rubbed the fleshy web between my thumb and index finger, noticing the bluish-purple marks still evident from where three-year-old Matthew Sims had sunk his teeth into it, refusing to let go until I cuffed him. Since that time he had idolized me and would allow no one else to work with him.

When Stirewalt came in, I pulled myself to a standing position, supporting my weight with my right leg. I worked my fingers nervously, gripping and regripping the worn wooden bars until Stirewalt grasped the waistband of my jeans. Then I shifted my weight to my arms, smashing the palms of my hands down against the bars as I brought my right leg up; extending the leg, I positioned my foot and pulled hard with my arms. My body inched forward until my leg was beneath me. I gradually allowed the leg to accept my weight. When it had, I leaned to my right and hiked my left hip. By pulling with my right arm while pushing with the left, I spun to the right, swinging the limp left leg forward. My toe caught the floor, jerking me off balance. My right knee buckled and I stumbled forward; fighting to hold myself up with my arms and pushing down hard with my right leg, I managed to lock my knee. I repositioned myself, but my left foot was still several inches behind me, so I hiked my hip again and spun to the right, jerking the leg forward. I worked my fingers around the bars, searching for a firmer grip before taking a second step.

Sweat was stinging my eyes, I was breathing heavily, and the overtaxed muscles of my arms and shoulders were beginning to swell from their grueling journey by the time I reached the end of the bars.

"Hold it here," Stirewalt told me. "I'll get the chair."

"I can make it back," I panted.

"I know you can, but it would be mostly by your arms. Your leg's had it, and besides I want to talk to you."

I eased myself into the chair and relaxed as Stirewalt pushed me to the staff lounge. He set a cup of coffee in front of me and seated himself across from me. He sat staring into his own cup as he rolled it back and forth between his hand.

"How long's it been now? Sixteen months?" he asked without looking up.

"Sixteen here, two in Asheville."

"Eighteen months," he mused. "A long time."

"You're telling me."

"If you were going to get any more return, we should have seen some signs of it by now, don't you think?" he asked, glancing up at me.

"I don't know." I shrugged. "You know as well as I do that return can come as late as five years after an accident."

"Sometimes," he conceded unwillingly in a subdued tone. "But it's usually spotty, and you can't wait five years before deciding which way to jump. You reach a point where you've got to go with what you've got, and right now—after sixteen months of therapy—what you've got is partial use of one leg. I think it's time we decided where we're going."

"What you got in mind?" I asked cautiously.

"Braces."

"What?" I was stunned. I couldn't believe he would even consider such a course.

"I'd like to try long leg braces."

I stared disbelievingly at him.

"Now just wait a minute," he said quickly before I could voice any protest. "I know. I know it's not what you were shooting for but . . . well, your legs aren't responding the way we hoped they would, and I thought that maybe, if we tried braces, even on a temporary basis . . ." He let his voice trail off and looked expectantly toward me.

I stiffened and the corners of my mouth turned down.

"I just feel that with braces we might be able to get you functional to a point—"

"To a point?" I snapped. "Swinging my legs like a polio victim is functional? Not to me it isn't."

"Tom, it'll allow you to be independent to a degree that—"

"I'm not interested in degrees," I argued. "It's got to be total. I've got to be totally independent when I leave here, and I can't do that if I start compromising now. Listen, I can beat this thing. Just hang on, don't quit on me now."

"It's been *eighteen* months; my God, you've pushed it as far as you can—as far as anybody could."

"No! No, I haven't." Desperation edged my words. "I can beat it, Stirewalt. Dammit man, I can win."

"You've already won! Don't you know that?" Stirewalt flared up angrily. "Goddammit boy, don't you know what you've done? You didn't have a prayer. When they rolled you in here the second time it was just to go through the motions. Nobody expected—"

"I expected!" I said through clenched teeth, jerking a thumb toward my chest. "I expected to do it and I still expect to do it."

"Don't you know that what you've done can't be done? The first time was a miracle, but this—" Stirewalt shook his head slowly. "There's nobody walking around out there that's been where you've been—*nobody*. And I'm not sure you can make it with braces, but we can give it one hell of a go."

"No," I said adamantly. "No braces. I won't need 'em."

The redness of Stirewalt's face deepened with anger.

"Listen you hardheaded son-of-a-bitch, we've got one month," he bellowed, leaning forward and holding a finger up to my face. "One goddamned lousy month and you're out. You're being discharged. One stinking month and I had to promise to walk on water to get that. They think a chair is it for you, but I held out for braces."

"Discharged?" I was stunned. "On whose order?"

"Walters'. Walters says you've had it. You've run your course."

"What the hell's he know. I haven't seen the son-of-a-bitch. He sends his flunkies."

"He gets weekly reports and he attends the conferences. You don't have to be a genius to see the lack of progress in the charts. And vocational rehab agrees with him. They're cutting off the money."

"Well, screw 'em. Vocational rehab was your idea, not mine. I didn't ask 'em for their money and—"

"No, you didn't ask them, but they've forked out to the tune of twenty thousand dollars, and when Walters says it's bought all it can—that's it. Now, we've got one month and I'm not sure you can manage braces— Are you listening to me?"

"I'll do it at home," I said, more to myself than to Stirewalt. "There are some old mattresses in the attic and—"

"Tom, for God's sake," he pleaded. "At least try it. You can still maintain an exercise program—hell, you'll have to."

"No," I said, looking at him soberly. "I can't. I can't start compromising. Not now."

"You won't even consider it?"

"I can't."

He turned his palms up, sighed, and shook his massive head in regretful disappointment; then he stood and walked out of the room.

I watched him go and felt an overwhelming sense of loss. The silence of the room bore an oppressive loneliness. Maybe it couldn't be done, I thought. Stirewalt's alliance had lent credence to my belief in myself, had strengthened my resolve and had made it seem possible, but now he was gone and with him all the needed tools. If I couldn't do it with Stirewalt and millions of dollars' worth of equipment, how could I possibly do it alone? Stirewalt was no fool. He wouldn't give up easily—he hadn't given up easily. He had hung in against all odds, and he would have bucked Walters if he had thought there was any hope at all. Maybe he was right. Maybe they were all right.

So what if they were? Those braces would always be there. I could pick them up anywhere along the line, and the quickest way for that to happen was to sit around wondering about myself.

What if my parents agreed with them? My father, maybe. But not Mom. She would never lose faith in me. She would be just as shocked by the idea as I had been, and just as determined to continue the struggle at home. It would have to be her idea though. She would have to suggest it. I could never ask them to accept that burden. I had decided that in Asheville. I would simply tell them what Stirewalt had told me, and if they suggested trying at home, okay. If not . . . I'd have to go with braces—for a while, anyway.

I pushed away from the table. Matthew Sims would be ex-

207

pecting me in the gym. Stirewalt was wrong. Vocational rehab was wrong. Dr. Walters was wrong. I could do it. I simply had to keep believing it, I told myself as I rolled out of the lounge.

I told my parents of Dr. Walters' decision the following Sunday as we sat in the lobby. Dad looked down at the floor and chewed the corner of his lip.

"How can they say you're not making progress?" Mom asked, staring at me in astonishment. "What about your arms? What about your left arm?"

"My arms are fine, they'll continue to improve with use. It's my legs. They think a wheelchair's the best I can do. Stirewalt thinks braces, maybe."

She stiffened. Her eyes narrowed and grew cold. Dad nodded solemnly. We sat that way—in silence—for a while.

"You say Stirewalt wants to try braces?" Dad asked with a frown. It was his habit to frown when he thought seriously about something.

"He's not sold on the idea, but he wants to try it."

"With braces you'd be able to give up the wheelchair completely?"

With averted eyes I nodded, trying not to show the disappointment I felt. My father could see only two alternatives, both of which led to a life I was not ready or willing to accept.

"You won't be giving up anything? You won't be losing anything? It will be a step forward?" Dad asked.

"I suppose so," I said.

"Compared to a wheelchair it should be—"

"You've told us what they say," Mom interrupted. "Now, what do you say?" Her voice carried with it a challenge.

"I think they're giving up too soon."

"It's not a matter of giving up, Tom," Dad put in. "I don't see how you can feel that moving from a wheelchair to braces is giving up."

"Stirewalt wouldn't have suggested braces unless he had

given up hope of my ever walking again," I explained.

"If you tried the braces, you could still work toward the day when you wouldn't need them, couldn't you?"

Mom looked at him and her face was worried.

"They're two different roads," I said. "I can't go both ways. Either one is going to require commitment. Braces aren't therapy. I can't put on braces hoping it will make my legs stronger."

"I didn't think about it that way," he said. "In fact, braces can actually make your legs weaker—doing the work for them, huh?"

"Yes. The less I use them . . ."

"Well, do you think—if we helped you—you could continue the exercises at home?"

"Yes," I said without hesitation.

Mom leaned over and kissed him on the cheek, and I knew that she had been waiting for him to make the suggestion just as eagerly as I had. And that if he hadn't made it she would. He looked at her, and his brow wrinkled in puzzlement at what had prompted the kiss.

I wanted to shout. I wanted to pick them both up and swing them around the room. I wasn't alone anymore. There was still a chance. No matter what anybody said, with or without Stirewalt, with or without Walters, with or without a million dollars' worth of equipment—there was still a chance. There was still hope.

"You realize that I won't be there during the day," he said to Mom, "and you'll end up with the lion's share of the work."

"I know," she said.

"Okay," he said to me, "what are we going to need?"

"Not much. Most of it you can pick up at a sporting goods store," I said. Then I looked at Mom. "I'm not going to lie to you, Mom. It's going to involve a lot of work. Six to eight hours a day. I can do most of it, but I need some help with a few of the exercises, and I'll need someone there most of the time to hand me weights."

"Well, I'm no Stirewalt"—she smiled—"but I try hard and I'm a fast learner."

"Is that old mattress still in the attic?"

"The twin mattress? Yes, I think so."

"Well, you'd better get it down and dust it off. I'm going to be spending a lot of time on it."

"What about bars?" Dad asked. "You're going to need parallel bars, aren't you?"

"Yes," I said thoughtfully. "Could you get somebody to come in and build me a set?"

"That shouldn't be much of a problem."

"Okay. How about running them along the wall from my bed to the bathroom."

"Okay, but what about the bathroom? You going to need anything special there? Rails?"

"No, I don't think so. I'll need a chair to set in the shower, but any ol' chair'll do. I'll make you a list of things to pick up and give it to you next Sunday, okay?"

"Okay, ace," he said, slapping his hands together. "By the time you get home we'll have it set up and ready to go." He slapped Mom on the knee and said, "Well, ol' girl, you ready to head for home? Maybe we'd better start you on an exercise program to get you ready." He winked at me.

Mom watched my face as she stood up.

"Don't look so worried," she said. Bending down she kissed me on the cheek and whispered, "I can remember another time when we were the only ones that thought you could do it." Straightening, she smiled down at me knowingly. "All the faith in the world in yourself and none in your mother, huh?"

"No, it's not that," I said awkwardly. "It's just—well, I'm not sure you realize just how much you're taking on."

"Stop worrying," she said as she crossed the room. Stopping, she looked back at me. Her eyes were mischievous. "You may have gotten your bullheadedness from your father, but that stubborn streak came directly from your mother. I can be just as stubborn as you, and I won't quit one minute before you do." She turned and they were gone.

I listened to the whispers of the empty lobby and the distant sounds of the hall. I started to tell myself once again that I could do it, but it wasn't necessary—I knew.

For the next two weeks I concentrated all of my effort toward improving my right leg. Neglecting all other exercises, I doubled and tripled the time on the parallel bars, soliciting the aid of one therapist after another when Stirwalt wasn't available. My hips and legs throbbed with a constant ache from the relentless, driving abuse. I pushed beyond fatigue and exhaustion, driving my body by force of will until at the end of the day I collapsed into bed glassy-eyed and sick to my stomach. And still my leg refused to respond, refused to improve. At the end of two weeks of torturous effort I could not take a single additional step.

When Stirewalt approached me, I was sitting on a padded table extending my leg against an aluminum bar from which weights were hung.

"Take five," he said.

I let my leg bend slowly beneath the pressure of the weights and looked at him.

"If you're going home in two weeks we'd better start teaching you a few things you're going to need to know," he said.

"Like what?" I asked, rubbing beads of sweat into the muscles of my leg with the heel of my hand.

"Like how to manage a few problems you're going to run into with a wheelchair. It's relatively simple around here, we're geared to it. Your bed raises and lowers, there are special showers and rails where you need them, and there aren't any cars in here for you to be climbing into. There are a few tricks I can show you that will make transferring into and out of that chair a hell of a lot easier."

I gripped the edges of the table and the muscles of my leg tightened, hardened, and shimmered beneath a film of sweat as I laboriously straightened my leg against the rattling protest of the weights. I held my breath and strained to keep my knee from bending.

"I'm not going to take a chair," I said, letting my breath out sparingly, almost a whisper.

"You're not what?" Stirewalt asked with surprise.

I looked back at my leg, watching the muscles shift and change as I let my knee bend gently beneath the weights.

"I'm not going to take a chair," I repeated.

"How the hell—you can't—" Stirewalt jerked his hands to his hips and stared down at the floor, shaking his head as if to clear it. "You can't walk," he explained indignantly. "You can't make it more than thirty feet in the *bars.*"

"That's far enough," I told him. "I've got bars from my bed to the bathroom. Thirty feet's far enough." I leaned forward on the table and rubbed the back of my neck. My neck always hurt when I sat unsupported.

"Look," Stirewalt said in a voice cracking with dismay, "when I suggested braces, I was buying time. You couldn't make it in braces, your hips aren't strong enough, but you can make it in a chair. You could—"

"I can't live in a chair," I said softly.

"If you go home like this you're gonna lose all we've gained. Six months at home and you won't be able to manage a chair. At least this way you've got a chance, you've got a shot at it."

"At what?" I asked.

"At life. At living a halfway decent life," he stormed.

"Halfway ain't good enough."

"Determination is one thing, but stupidity is another," he growled. His lips tightened and his eyes grew fierce. "And I've just about had it with you. A lot of people have put in a hell of a lot of effort to get you this far and—"

"You think it's easy?" I said with quick, flaring anger. "You think it's easy to say no to that chair? Every time I stand up

212

I get so scared I could puke. It's like somebody has his hand in my gut squeezing. Every time I come up on these legs I wonder if it's the last time. I wonder if I'll ever have the guts to try it again. A fall put me here and a fall can do it again and I'm scared of falling—I'm so goddamned scared I'm sick. Yeah, I'd like to take that chair home, you bet your sweet ass I would. I'd like to grab it and hold on and never have to feel that fear again, but I—" I stopped. Blood pounded at my temples. "I can't *live* in a chair. Once I sit down, a thousand doors slam shut."

"You still don't see it, do you? You're looking at it from the wrong side. Sure, if we told a normal person he was going to have to spend the rest of his life in a wheelchair, we'd be closing some doors. But offer it to a quad and you're offering him a miracle. You're opening a thousand doors. You're offering him life. And that's what you are, hot shot—a quad."

"Well, there it is," I said with an air of regret. "That's the difference in you and me. You're looking at it from a quad's point of view, and I'm looking at it from the way I used to be because that's the only way I can look at it. If I had accepted the fact that I was going to be a quad forever, then I would have welcomed life in a wheelchair. But I never reached that point—I never accepted it as final, as permanent."

"Well, you've reached that point now and the sooner—"

"No, you've reached it—I haven't."

"Tom, you're going to have to accept the fact that *this is it* for you. And you might as well do it now."

"No, I don't have to do it now. What's so goddamn magical about *now!* Because you and a bunch of doctors want to throw in the towel? Okay, okay, you may be right, but I'll pick my own time to hang it up, and it won't be until I *know* it won't do any good to pull myself out of that chair for one more try. When *I* know—I—*me*—when I know."

"Well, I've said all I can. I think you're wrong. I think you're making a mistake, a mistake you're going to regret." He looked

213

down at me, started to say something, then closed his mouth and walked away.

I watched him go, then stared down at my leg accusingly. With a sudden violent thrust I kicked my foot forward, straightening my leg with a force that spun the weights crazily on the aluminum bar and sent one crashing noisily to the floor. I sat holding the leg rigid, glaring at it with cold contempt, viciously jerking my knee back into position, punishing it each time it began to buckle beneath the weight.

During the next two weeks, Stirewalt devoted more time than ever to me, but he kept the relationship strictly professional—almost cold. He spent the last rush of days acting more as an instructor than a therapist, suggesting various substitutes for the equipment in the gym, explaining why it was important for one particular exercise to follow another, pointing out again and again exactly what Mom was to do, how she was to stand, where she was to place her hand, how much resistance she was to apply, and making me repeat the instructions time after time until he was sure there would be no mistake. But he brought no enthusiasm to the task—there was none of the old rivalry or the constant, challenging banter that had characterized our relationship. We did not look at each other during the awkward silences when each searched for words neither was able to find. And so the last workday passed as the one before it—with words left unspoken, with good-byes left unsaid.

Now as I lay on my bed waiting for my parents to come, I ran a finger over the braided edges of a small purse and watched a sad-faced Althea Biggers expertly maneuver her small wheelchair toward the door. Although I had said my good-byes the previous evening, Althea had come to bring a yellow and green change purse she had made for me in occupational therapy.

Mom almost tripped over her as she and Dad came into the room.

"You must be Althea," she said.

"Yes, ma'am," Althea answered without looking up.

"Well, I'm so glad I finally got to meet you. Tom's told us so much about you."

"Are you his mother?" she asked.

"Yes."

"Well, he's the meanest person I ever met," she said petulantly, her large brown eyes filling with tears.

Mom smiled down at her with understanding.

"But I still love him," she said defiantly, her tiny voice beginning to crack.

Mom looked at her tenderly, then she knelt down and took her by the hand.

"I love him too," she whispered. "But sometimes he makes it awfully difficult."

Althea wiped at her nose with the back of her hand and sniffed.

"I'll tell you what," Mom said, standing. "Why don't I take you back to your room? I think the boys can manage without us."

She nodded to Dad and disappeared into the hall.

"You 'bout ready to go home, boy?" he asked.

"Thought you'd never get here," I told him.

"I'll run these out to the car," he said, picking up the bags. "Then I've got to stop by the office and sign you out."

"I'll meet you in the lobby," I told him.

I tucked the change purse into my shirt pocket and transferred from the bed to a wheelchair. I checked the bedside cabinet and the dresser drawers once again to see that nothing had been forgotten. As I turned to leave, Stirewalt stepped into the room.

"You gonna leave without saying good-bye?" he asked.

"I had to pass the gym on my way out," I said without expression.

"I'm right. Everything I've said is right," he explained

215

harshly. "I know it. So tell me why I feel like a damn deserter, huh?"

I smiled and shrugged.

"I made you a list of exercises and I brought you a little going-home present," he said, tossing two red and white objects into my lap.

"What—"

"Knee pads," he explained. "I was thinking about it last night and it hit me—crawling. We tried it earlier, remember?"

"I remember," I said cautiously.

"Your left hip wouldn't support you. Your left shoulder wasn't much good at that time either, but it's come along—so—maybe—if you concentrate on the right exercises—"

"You want me to crawl?"

"What's the matter? You don't like the idea? You too good to crawl? Babies crawl, don't they? Why the hell ya think babies crawl?"

I shrugged.

"To build the muscles necessary for walking," he explained. "And that's what you've got to do. Forget the bars. Forget trying to walk. If we can get that left hip strong enough to support you crawling, that will work on the same muscles. Once they're strong enough, then you can use the bars to work on coordination and balance. Look," he said, excitedly jerking a piece of paper from his hip pocket, "I've marked the exercises I want you to concentrate on. Number eight," he said, holding the paper down to me and pointing to it, "and number eleven and seventeen and—well, you can see, I've marked 'em, and I've written in the number of repetitions and the amount of weight. Now when—as soon as you can, I want you to start crawling. I mean, I want you to wear those pads down to the threads. You can't over—"

I turned slowly and gazed up at him with a sly grin.

He looked at me steadily for a moment.

216

"This doesn't mean I think you can pull it off," he explained indignantly. "I don't."

"Oh?"

"No. I just think that if there's any possibility at all, this is it."

"I see."

"All you would have accomplished in the bars would have been a lousy walking pattern for the few feet you managed to drag yourself. Not even you can develop a bad crawling pattern."

"Is that a fact?"

"Yes, it's a fact," he snapped smugly. "And I still say it can't be done."

"I'll do it."

"No way."

"Cup of coffee says I will."

"You're on, hard nose. Stay in touch," he said over his shoulder as he walked out of the room.

19

I winced against a sudden prick of pain as the worn leather strap bit into the tender flesh of my ankle, causing my leg to jerk involuntarily. The heavy lead weights hanging from the strap thudded together dully and jerked at their fastenings. I ignored the growing pain in my ankle and forced the throbbing muscles of my hip to hold my leg suspended until the weights were motionless. Lying on my right side with my left leg raised, watching the weights for any sign of movement, I finished a long, slow count and continued to hold my leg rigid until the burning protest of muscle could no longer be ignored. Then I lowered my leg and rolled onto my back. I was glad the weights had not moved. If they had, I would have had to repeat the exercise. It was a game I played—one of many—to make the endless hours of exercise less boring. But I was especially pleased not to have to repeat this particular exercise because it was the last one I intended to do.

Sitting up, I unbuckled the ankle strap and set it along with the lead weights to one side, but there was no air of celebration in the final putting away of tools whose use I so deplored. There was no joy or sense of victory in the act. The realization

218

had not come easily or quickly, but it had come; I would walk with a cane for the rest of my life. No amount of effort or time would change that. No amount of exercise or anger could wrest anything further from a besieged body.

For over two years I had driven doggedly through a mounting hatred for the interminable exercises. Sweating and straining, fighting to get above the pain, day after day, with no holiday and no rest, I had cajoled and harassed and coerced languid muscles into response, into movement, into life. I had worn out one set of knee pads after another until I had lost count of their number. I had dragged myself through the parallel bars until their rough wood was worn smooth and gleamed with a polished finish born from the sweat of callused hands. It had taken me more than two years, but I had gone from crawling, to crutches, to canes, and finally to a single cane.

And now I wondered if I had won or lost. I would never again beat Rick in a game of tennis or feel the power of my legs as I drove over Wayne in a game of one on one. I would never be able to walk in the sand of a beach or across a snow-covered field. I wouldn't carry out the garbage or stand in a chair to change a light bulb. I would never dance again or run again. I would never mow the grass again or rake the leaves again or clip the hedges or wash the car or paint the house. There were a thousand things I would never do again, but most of them would have been left behind in time anyway, I told myself. For most of the men I know, the golf course was the most physical arena they entered. They didn't ski or play tennis or frolic in the snow or dance. And they didn't mow the grass—not if they could pay someone to do it for them. The only time they walked on a beach was to go from a lounge to a cooler for another beer. I'd never seen my father run, didn't even know if he could run. No, I wasn't losing that much; time would have robbed me of most of it anyway.

I heard Wayne's voice from somewhere in the house. He was home from college for the summer. Jesus, it was hard to believe that Wayne had finished his second year of college. It always surprised me to realize that time had not stopped for everyone the way it had for me. I reached for the edge of the bed and pulled myself to my feet. I had lost four years and this bothered me more than the prospect of living with a cane. I had catching up to do. I was in a hurry to get back into the rhythm of life, to feel its ebb and flow, to be a part of it again. Okay, maybe I was rationalizing about what I had lost, but the one thing I had not lost, the one thing four years of uncompromising effort had won for me, was a chance at life. I could still have everything I wanted, everything I had prepared for, everything I had waited for.

I moved along the edge of the bed until I could reach the cane propped against the desk. I picked it up, and as I turned I looked back at the telephone. I hesitated for a moment— unsure. I had to start somewhere, I told myself. If I was positive that I had come as far as I could physically, and if I was going to put my life back together, there was no better place to start than Cory.

I sat down and picked up the receiver. I didn't expect her to be there, not after four years, but I had promised myself that I would make the call. I started to dial but couldn't remember the number, and that surprised me. It was the one number I thought I would never forget. Opening the desk drawer, I took out my wallet and found the number, dialed it and waited. Cory's mother answered on the third ring.

"Mrs. Benton, this is Tom Helms. May I speak to Cory?"

There was an awkward silence.

"Tom, how nice. Where are you?" Her voice just missed the pleasant surprise it was intended to convey.

"I'm at home. Could—"

"Well, how are you getting along?"

"Fine, I'm fine."

"Are you walking now? The last we heard . . ."

She knew! But how could she know? And if Cory knew,

why hadn't she called? I started to ask but decided not to. I would find out from Cory.

"Yes, I'm walking. I'm doing quite well, thank you. Could you tell me how to reach Cory?"

"You should have let us know. We didn't find out until about a year ago. Cory ran into one of your fraternity brothers. You should have let us know."

"I know," I said apologetically. Damn that tone. I hated that tone and I always ended up using it with her. "Where is Cory now?"

"She's in Atlanta."

"Could you give me her number?"

There was another silence.

"She's married, Tom. She was married almost a year ago."

I couldn't think of anything to say. I wasn't surprised. I just didn't have anything to say.

"In fact," she said, when it became evident that I was not going to reply, "it was at her wedding that she found out you had been in the hospital."

Well, that explained why she didn't call, I thought.

"She married a very nice young man from here in Savannah," she continued. "He's in his last year of residency in Atlanta, and they seem to be very happy."

And I know you are, I started to say, but didn't. I had had my confrontation with Mrs. Benton, although indirectly, and had come away the loser. Nothing could be gained by an angry exchange now. But, damn her, she had to get in that residency bit, didn't she?

"I hope she's happy," I said. "I hope they'll both be happy. Tell her I called the next time you see her, and give her my best wishes."

I hung up the phone and sat staring at it, trying to understand my emotions—or rather, my lack of emotion. I was relieved. The only thing I felt was relief, and I wondered why. I had known she wouldn't be there. I had known it from the first

221

lucid moment following surgery. I knew it then, and if not then, certainly in the long slow months that followed. Four years was a long time, and somewhere in those years the pain of losing Cory had melted into physical pain until recovery from one was recovery from both. Somewhere in those years I had lost Cory Benton, but I didn't know where, I couldn't remember the moment or the day. The days had a sameness that was smothering, that numbed emotion and dulled desire.

But why relief? Why feel relieved? I had loved Cory, and it didn't make sense that I should be relieved, almost glad, she was no longer in my life. I had dreaded making that call, had put it off for days, and now I knew it wasn't the fear of finding that Cory was lost to me forever, but fear of finding that she wasn't. I had walked out of her life, and if I was ever to enter it again it would be with a limp, leaning on a cane. I didn't want to go back like that. I didn't want to try to put together the pieces of a past that could not be reconstructed. Maybe in time, with effort, we might have rediscovered each other, but it would never have been the same because I wasn't the same. There would have always been the memories of other days, the comparisons, the wistful wonderings of what our life might have been had it been allowed to continue as it had started. No, I was glad I didn't have to face that, and I was glad I didn't have to see the expression on her face the first time she saw me.

I thought of the two small moles on her left temple and wondered why they should come to mind. I had noticed them the first day we met as she sat across from me in that little coffee shop. I couldn't remember seeing them again during the time we had gone together. Maybe her hair covered them or maybe I just hadn't noticed them again, but it was odd that I should remember them now. Maybe a poet could make something of it, or a philosopher, but I was neither and I was in a hurry, I had catching up to do. There would be another girl in my life, someday—if my life was to have any meaning.

I stood up slowly and stiffly and reached for the cane. As I stepped forward on my right foot, my left foot turned in and the heel came off the floor. I swung my left leg forward in an arc, the toes barely clearing the floor. When I placed my foot back on the floor my toes touched first and my leg trembled as I fought the spasms to force the heel flush against the floor. I was fortunate that the spasticity was limited to the left leg and that it was no more severe than it was. But still it was the spasticity that bound me to a cane, that wrecked my balance and destroyed the pattern. I hated the way I walked, the sound of my left foot scraping the floor when I was too tired to clear it, the tremors that greeted me with each step, the halting, staggering attempt to regain a lost balance. But at least it was walking, I told myself as I made my way down the hall, and as long as I could think of my body as a vehicle that transported me from one place to another, then it served its purpose.

"Where are my car keys?" I asked, coming into the den.

My mother and brother exchanged looks. I had not been out of the house in two years except for an occasional ride with Wayne or my father.

"Why?" Mom asked.

"My license has expired, and I think I better find out if I can drive before I try to renew it."

"You think you're ready for that?" Wayne asked.

"I'd better be."

"You're sure?" Mom asked.

I looked at her and knew she wasn't referring to driving.

"Yes. I've gone as far as I can."

"You don't think that a few more months—"

"No, Mom. And if you'll be honest you don't think so either."

"Maybe you're right. Maybe getting back into the activity of everyday living will do more good than all the exercises. Your keys are on the bar."

"Wait a minute!" Wayne said. "You haven't driven in four years. You just can't . . . what if you have a spasm?"

I glanced at Mom and saw the smile. Wayne made no distinction between the slight tremors in my left leg and the violent eruptions he had witnessed in other patients during his visits to the hospital. To his way of thinking, one could always precipitate the other.

"Hang on and ride it out, I guess," I told him. "You've kept my car in good running order, haven't you?"

"Yes, but—"

"Then there's nothing to worry about."

"Mom," Wayne pleaded.

"Why don't you go with him, Wayne?"

"Me?"

"That's right, hot shot. Why don't you come along? It might be a ride to remember."

He considered it for a moment then said, "All right, but I'll drive. We'll find a safe spot and then you can give it a try."

"What you got in mind, the middle of an empty parking lot?" I laughed as Wayne picked up the keys and headed for the door.

Mom raised her eyebrows and pointed a finger of warning at me as I followed Wayne out the door. I winked at her and pulled the door closed behind me.

I shifted the cane to my left hand and grasped the rail with my right. I was glad my father had installed the rail, because steps were going to be a problem. I had to step forward onto my left leg because I could not trust it to support my weight and lower me to the next step. As I lowered myself with my right leg, the toes of my left foot touched the step first and the struggle to force the heel down began. When my foot was placed firmly, I brought my right leg down beside it and repeated the process one step at a time until I reached the driveway. It was slow, but no real problem as long as there was a rail. I wasn't sure I could manage without one. The spasticity often threw me off balance, and it was a simple matter to place the cane either in front or behind me to correct the loss and keep from falling. This would not be possible on steps. If I lost my balance forward, the only surface upon which I could place the cane would be a lower step. I would have to lean even farther forward to accomplish this, and the result would be falling face first down the steps. If I lost my balance backward and managed to position the cane on a step above and behind me, the positioning would make it impossible to derive the necessary support from the cane. But I would probably not fall backward. The spasticity pulled my foot down, which pitched me forward. If I was going to fall, it would more than likely be down the steps.

Damn the luck, I thought as I climbed into the car. People get killed falling down stairs. Hell, I had already broken my neck falling down stairs—not even stairs, just a few lousy steps. You were always reading in the paper where some old lady or some old man had taken a tumble down a flight of stairs and died. You never read about anybody falling *up* the stairs and doing themselves in, or falling backward on the stairs. The little bit of spasticity I had just had to be the kind that might one day kill me. Damn!

"I don't know why you're in such a hurry," Wayne said as he backed the car out of the drive. "All of a sudden, right out of the blue, wham, you've got to start driving. It's got to be today. Well, I think you're rushing it. I think you ought to take it a little at a time."

"Okay," I agreed jokingly. "Today I'll sit in your lap and steer. You can work the pedals until I learn to guide the thing."

"Be serious."

"I am serious."

He made a face.

"How do you learn to drive a little at a time, huh? I'm not learning—I know how. I just want to check my reaction time, to get the feel of it again. What do you suggest we do? Stay in the back yard and practice going forward and backing up?"

"Hell, no." He laughed. "What if you have a spasm and it presses your foot down the way it does? We got two choices—

slam into the bank or slam into the house. No, sir, I'm going to get you out in the wide open spaces where we've got room for error."

As he backed the car down the drive I remembered another time we had gone down that drive together. It was almost a year earlier, during Wayne's freshman year. He was home for a weekend and had bought a new motorcycle. I had just learned to take a few halting steps with crutches and he insisted that I come out to see his new bike. It was easier for me to get out the front of the house, so he pulled the bike around to the front yard, and as we stood looking at it the pride in his eyes turned into devilment.

"Let's go for a ride," he said, as if he were proposing the violation of some sacred law, and a slow grin crawled across his face.

"What?" I asked with astonishment.

"I'll go slow." He nodded with a smile and promise. "Come on. It'll be good for you. How long's it been since you've been on a bike?"

"Not as long as it's going to be," I said, leaning heavily on the crutches and beginning to have serious doubts as to whether I had the strength to make it back to the house.

"Aw, come on," he said, and a look of disappointment crossed his face.

I looked at him with an uncertain grin.

"I'll hold it and you get on," he suggested eagerly.

I thought about it and knew I didn't have the strength to get back to the house. My knees were beginning to buckle and I was so tired I just wanted to sit down. The bike was the nearest seat.

"Okay," I told him.

He held the bike and I was able, by using the crutches and coming up on tiptoes, to inch my way over the rear fender and onto the seat. I tossed the crutches to one side and used my hands to position my feet on the stirrups.

226

"Hold on," he said as he gently shoved the bike into motion. We went around the house and down the drive. My foot bounced off the stirrup when we hit the bump at the end of the drive, and he had to stop while I repositioned it. The vibrations of the motor kept shimmying my foot off the stirrup, so we tried riding with me holding one leg out to the side, but I tired quickly so we headed back home.

Wayne pulled the bike up beside the crutches and we sat there for a minute.

"Well?" he finally said.

"Well what?"

"Well, get off."

"How?"

He thought for a minute and then said, "Can you stand there and let me drive it out from under you?"

"No, my legs aren't long enough."

"Come up on your toes."

"And fall on my face?"

"Can you reach your crutches?"

"Can you?"

"No." He chuckled. "Can you stand on one leg and hold the other up?"

"It's all I can do to stand on both legs and crutches."

"Well, can you hold the bike if I get off and get the crutches?"

"Be serious. I'm gonna hold up a bike when I can't even stand?"

"Well, we gotta do something quick, Mom's due back any minute and if she sees this . . ."

"Can you run the thing up there between the shrubbery and the house? I could grab one of those bushes—"

"Mom will kill me if I run over her shrubbery."

"Well, she'll go into cardiac arrest if she catches me on this damn motorcycle," I said. "This is just about the dumbest idea you ever had."

"You didn't have to get on."

"No, but I've got to get off, don't I?"

"You got any ideas?"

"We can't do it alone. We need someone to hand me the crutches, so we flag down a car."

"I ain't gonna flag down no car. That's embarrassing."

"We don't have any choice, so pull it down there beside the street."

He grumbled as he moved the bike and again as I whistled and waved at passing cars. Finally a car pulled over to the curb and a man asked if there was any trouble.

"I wonder if you'd mind handing us those crutches up there in the yard," I said.

He looked at our legs and didn't see a cast. Then he just sat there and grinned at us like we were trying to pull something and he had our number. Wayne turned red and hung his head.

"I can't walk without crutches," I explained.

"How'd you get on then?"

"I had the crutches when I got on."

He looked at me, not sure whether to believe me or not. Wayne was crimson.

"If you guys are putting me on . . ." he had said, getting out of the car.

Now as Wayne and I drove out of town in the car the road curved down a gentle hill and stretched out level and flat for more than a mile before it twisted into a sharp curve. Wayne pulled off to the side of the road and said, "This is as good a place as any."

"This is where I brought you when I first taught you to drive," I said.

"History does have a way of repeating itself, doesn't it." He smiled smugly.

"I guess," I replied. "I suppose the next thing is for you to have a talk with me about sex."

"What would you like to know?"

"You mean you've learned something since we had our little talk?"

"No, but I've added a few innovations of my own that you might find interesting," he said, getting out of the car.

"I'll bet you have." I chuckled as I slid over behind the wheel. "How come you had that talk with me anyhow? I always expected the old man to do that."

"He told me he thought it was time you knew the facts of life and that he wanted me to have a little talk with you," I explained, as I checked the movement of my foot from the gas pedal to the brake. I was pleased with the speed with which I could make the move and glad that the car was an automatic and that my left leg was not needed.

"Why didn't he do it?"

"I don't know. I told him that I thought it was his job but he refused. Said if you were going to find out it was up to me."

"Did he ever have a talk with you?"

"Hell, no. Not a word. I learned it in the street like everybody else. Are you ready to give it a go?" I said, buckling the seat belt and shifting the selector to drive.

"Wait a minute," he said, hunting for his seat belt. "Now listen—take it slow and easy, and if you think you're going to have a spasm, don't pull off the road. Just try to get your foot off the gas."

I stared disbelievingly at him.

"If you pull off the road with your foot on the floor, we're going to lose it for sure," he explained.

"I see," I said, and I started to punch the gas pedal and yell "spasm" just to watch him jump, but I decided not to. That's what Mom's warning had been all about.

"And if you have—"

I pulled the car onto the road and let the speed steadily increase until we reached the posted limit, then I turned and grinned at him with a superior smirk.

229

He looked at me with dawning comprehension. "You don't have any spasticity in your right foot, do you?"

"Nope."

"Why didn't you say so?"

"You didn't ask."

We were quiet as we rode for a while through rolling hills and farm country. I'd forgotten how beautiful a summer day could be.

Finally I turned the car toward home and my thoughts toward the coming week. I had been reading the want ads for the past few days, and there were several I hoped to answer. It wasn't going to be a simple matter of going on an interview. It was going to be my baptism under fire, the first real test of how well I could function in the world.

I was going to have to seek employment in Charlotte because there was none in Concord, except the mills, and I had sworn never to work in the mills. I had inherited a hatred for the textile mills from my mother, who had watched them suck the life out of her mother and father.

I wondered exactly what it was the mills did to the people and why. I supposed it had something to do with the destruction of the spirit. It was evident on their faces and in their manner. Maybe it was because no decisions were left to them, no choices.

The last significant decision most of them made came with high-school graduation. They either chose to work in the mills or to leave town by going to college or entering military service. Those who left rarely came back for more than a brief visit with their parents.

I had chosen to leave, and I was back through no choice of my own, but I wasn't driven back as some had been. I wasn't retreating from a hostile world, seeking the numbing womb of the mill. I was on my way out again.

20

THE following week I threaded the car through downtown traffic, looking for the building in which I had an interview. I had taken the driver's exam two days earlier, and the only restriction it carried limited me to cars with automatic transmissions. Since they were the only ones I could drive, the necessity of noting it on the license seemed ridiculous.

I found the building I was looking for and was relieved to find a parking lot half a block away. It was on the opposite side of the street, though, and I dreaded crossing those four lanes. I paid the attendant and parked the car. I stepped out and straightened my pants and adjusted my coat. The coat was a little loose across the shoulders, but the pants had been altered to compensate for the twenty pounds I had lost since purchasing the blue pin-striped suit just prior to graduation.

As I walked down the sidewalk toward the traffic signal, I was surprised, almost shocked, at how different I felt. At home I felt completely normal, and there was no need to be concerned as to whether or not the cane would hold. I knew the surfaces of the house intimately; there was always a wall or a chair or a door to catch a quick, jabbing elbow and aid me

231

in regaining a lost balance. Here there were no walls, and the surfaces were unfamiliar, requiring me to test them before committing myself to the cane. I had to look at each spot where I intended to place the cane or my foot. A pebble could roll beneath the tip of the cane; a rock accidentally stepped on could cost me my precarious balance. The fraction of an inch I was able to clear my left foot had been sufficient on the smooth floors of my parents' house, but sidewalks were not smooth; there were ridges and cracks and padding for expansion. I had to slow my pace and make an extra effort upon each encounter with obstacles invisible to those hurrying by me. That surprised me, too—the speed with which everybody moved. I seemed hopelessly out of step with everything around me. I smiled at the thought, pleased with how appropriate the choice of phrases was. I *was* out of step, but the race I was running would not necessarily go to the swift.

I noticed the quick, darting glances of those I met. Nothing obvious, just a dropping of the eyes for a quick look at my legs. That wasn't what bothered me. It was natural for them to look, I supposed. It was that final searching look from my legs back to my face that began to arouse the first twinges of resentment. What did they hope to find reflected in my face? An evil, perhaps? Something so vile that it would justify any amount of carnage wrought upon me? Or maybe they hoped to find a calm acceptance which would grant them absolution for their normalcy. Maybe they expected bitterness or a compassionate wisdom born of trial. Whatever they sought, they would not find it in the chiseled features of an expressionless face. I looked down at the sidewalk, thankful for an excuse not to have to meet their stares.

I stood on the corner waiting for the light to change. I would have to commit my entire weight to my left leg and the cane as I came off the curb. If my knee buckled, I would go down, and I shuddered at the thought. If I fell I wouldn't be able to get up. I had tried it on the floor of the bedroom. It was

232

impossible unless there was something upon which I could use my arms, something upon which I could pull. If I fell, I would try to fall near a car, I decided. I paled at the thought of lying helpless in the middle of a busy street. The only thing worse would be to fall down steps, I thought, with a quick look down the block at my intended destination. No steps. Thank God for small favors.

The light changed, and I brought my left leg up hurriedly and immediately lost my balance. I jammed the cane to one side and steadied myself. I repositioned my feet and slid my left foot forward without lifting it from the ground. I let the heel ride down against the curb as I lowered my foot. The contact helped me keep my balance. Just before my foot touched the gutter, I brought the cane down beside it to absorb part of my weight. My knee gave slightly, but I managed to lock it. I followed with the right foot, steadied myself, and stepped forward into the street. I had used too much time getting off the curb, I knew, but if I hurried maybe I could make it. I was less than halfway across when I heard the sickening click of the light changing. I heard the engines spring to life and just as quickly die. They would wait. They would wait and they would watch. I could feel them watching and I could feel the hot flush of embarrassment flood my face. I kept my head down, watching the pavement for that one spot of oil that would send the cane skidding out from under me, and tried desperately to hurry. I brought my left foot forward too fast and failed to clear it. My toe jammed against the pavement and I staggered forward, turning sideways, fighting for balance. I could almost hear them gasp. God, I wished I could disappear. There was no telling who was in those cars, and they were all embarrassed, and in pain for me, and hoping I'd make it, and thinking what a terrible thing it was for such a young man to be in such terrible condition—and I wished I could disappear.

I reached the opposite curb and stopped, positioned my feet

233

for the step up, and then I became aware of the silence. There was no rush of engines. I was out of their way but no one was roaring away from the light. Jesus! They were watching. Waiting and watching. I brought my right foot up, placed it on the curb and, in one fluid movement, followed it with my left. I felt a great affection for my right leg; it had never failed me. In all I had been through, my right leg had never failed me, and no one watching from the waiting cars would ever be as proud of anything as I was of that single perfect step from the street to the curb.

I could feel the perspiration at my temples and across my forehead as I made my way the remaining distance down the block. I had it all to do over again, I thought as I entered the building. I had to cross that street again; I had to go through the humiliation all over again.

I found the office I was seeking, straightened my tie, wiped the sweat off my face, and stepped inside.

"I'm Tom Helms," I told the secretary. "I have a ten o'clock appointment with Mr. Billings."

She checked her calendar and nodded.

"Yes, would you fill this out, please," she said, handing me an application. "Mr. Billings will be with you in a moment."

I completed the application, returned it to the secretary, and waited.

I had almost fallen down back there in the street, I thought. If I pushed it going back, I probably would fall. But if I didn't push, if I didn't hurry . . .

"Mr. Helms? I'm Leonard Billings. Would you come in, please."

I struggled to rise from the low couch and silently cursed modern furniture. I didn't hurry as I started across the room. I had learned that the first four or five steps were the most difficult and the most awkward. Once I was able to establish a gait, my pattern would become smooth, more rhythmic, and

I could move faster with less effort. But, unfortunately, the initial impression would be conveyed during those first few steps.

I stopped in front of the man, shifted the cane to my left hand, and extended my right. When we shook hands, Mr. Billings exerted no pressure at all. He simply extended a limp hand, and I wondered if it was his normal handshake or if he purposely refrained from using any grip out of fear of hurting me.

"Come in and have a seat," Mr. Billings said. "Just give me a moment to look over your application."

I seated myself across the desk from him and watched as he read down the application. When he came to the space marked DO YOU HAVE ANY PHYSICAL HANDICAPS? where I had written "walk with a cane," he began asking about what I could and couldn't do physically and what had happened to make the use of a cane necessary. When he satisfied himself about my medical history, he told me the position had been filled earlier that morning. I was glad. I was relieved that I wouldn't have to cross that street in rush-hour traffic every morning.

"There's a strong possibility that something will be opening up in the near future, and I'll certainly keep you in mind when it does," he said.

I thanked him and left. I took my time crossing the street. No one was going to run over me as long as they could see me. My only real fear was that someone turning the corner wouldn't see me.

I killed an hour riding around, ate a slow lunch, and went on my second interview at one o'clock. They were looking for someone with more experience, but there was a chance that another job, requiring less experience, would be available soon.

It was a relief to get home. I hadn't relaxed since I left that morning. It was good to feel safe again, to be on surfaces I was familiar with, to be away from the stares and the crowds that moved so much faster than I.

Wayne kept shooting nervous glances at Mom when I told them about the interviews, and he kept looking at me with a silly grin tugging at the corners of his mouth.

"Are you very tired?" he finally asked.

"No, why?"

He grinned at Mom.

I looked at her suspiciously.

"You better tell him," she said. "He has to know before this evening anyway."

"Okay," he said, rubbing his hands together. "Are you ready for this, boy?"

"Probably not, but go ahead."

"You've got a date tonight."

I just stared at him. I was sure it was a joke and I waited for the kicker.

"It's true. You've got a date. Janice fixed it up."

"Who's Janice?"

"You know Janice. The girl I've been dating. Her older sister is home for a few days, and you've got a date with her."

"No, I don't," I told him. I didn't want a date. I hadn't planned to start dating yet. I hadn't even found out what I could or couldn't do yet. That street had surprised me. I hadn't thought crossing a street would be a problem. What else was out there waiting to surprise me? Whatever it was, I didn't want some girl I didn't even know along when I had to face it.

"Yes, you do," he insisted.

"I'm not going," I said flatly.

"You are so. You've got to go. Janice will kill me if you don't."

"You go. I'm staying home."

"Mom," he pleaded.

"It might be good for you," she said.

"It won't be good for me. I took a vow of celibacy."

"She's not that kind of girl," he argued.

"Then why would I want to go out with her?"

"Momma," he pleaded again.

"It won't hurt you to see the girl, just this once," she said.

"Don't you see what he's doing?" I asked. "His little girl friend's sister—who's probably a real snake—is bored, so Lochinvar there volunteers me."

"I did not! I'm trying to do you a favor. You're the one that's in such a hurry to get going again. I'm just trying to help you get a social life started."

"Sure you are."

He checked and made sure Mom wasn't looking at him. Then he made a threatening face at me which said that if I didn't go Janice would cut him off.

"I don't have any money," I told him.

"You don't need money," he said eagerly. "It's not a date date. You're just going to stop by for a drink. The family is going to be out for the evening. She'll be there all alone," he said, flicking his eyebrows up and down and then glancing quickly to see if Mom had seen.

I wasn't tired and I didn't have anything else to do. I didn't want to go because I didn't want to leave the safety of the house. I didn't want to face all the obstacles out there. I didn't want any more surprises. I wanted to hang on to the safety of the house, just as I had wanted to hang on to the safety of a wheelchair when Stirewalt had offered it. And that's why I had to go. I couldn't start hiding. My very first day back in the real world—and all I wanted to do was get back home.

"Okay," I said. "I'll go. But you owe me for this one, buster."

"My honor, my fortune, and my life—they're yours."

"You have no honor . . . or fortune, and if she turns out to be a dog, I wouldn't bet too much on your life."

It was raining when I left the house, and a raincoat that had fit four years earlier hung on me like a tent. I wondered if Wayne had told her I walked with a cane. I had forgotten to ask. Knowing him, probably not. At least I wouldn't have to cross any streets or climb any steps. Wayne had sworn there were no steps. I wondered if there were any throw rugs or waxed floors. I wondered if she had a concrete walk or a slate walk. I didn't think my cane would hold on slate. I wondered if . . .

I found the house and turned into the driveway. My headlights hit the house. *Steps!* Damn Wayne! There must be fifty steps and no rail. It looked like the stairway to heaven. How was I going to get up there? Getting up wasn't the problem. How the hell was I going to get down? And he swore there were no steps. Looked me in the eye and swore on his life.

I sat in the car and thought about going back home. But I couldn't avoid steps and streets and throw rugs forever. I'd just ask her to let me take her arm coming down the steps. It might be embarrassing, but there wasn't anything else I could do.

The walk was cement and so were the steps. I took them one at a time—stepping up with my right foot and then bringing my left foot up beside it. It was slow and by the time I reached the door I was soaked.

When she came to the door I knew why I had stopped going on blind dates when I was fifteen, and from her expression she wasn't any too pleased with me. How could she be? God only knew what she was expecting. Wayne had probably told her I was the spitting image of Paul Newman or something, and there I stood in a tent looking like a dead rat with my hair dripping water down my face.

Well, we're stuck with each other for the next few hours, I thought, try to make the best of it. I tried to be interesting and witty but her "yes," "no," and "I don't know" responses left time hanging in the air like a bad odor.

She had all the charm of a rock, and I knew it would be impossible for me to ask her to help me down those steps. The pauses in conversation grew longer and longer because

238

I kept trying to figure out how to manage those steps. Finally I decided that the only way to do it was to get out there and do it. I'd have to come up with something once I was standing at the top of them.

I suggested cutting the evening short because the weather was so bad. It didn't make much sense since we were inside and had no plans for going out, but she didn't seem to notice.

"There's no need for you to stand here in the damp," I said when we reached the door. "I'm pretty slow on steps. So why don't you just run on back in."

When she closed the door I stood there a moment to make sure she wasn't coming back. When I was sure she had gone to another part of the house, I took a deep breath, turned around, and fell off the porch.

I landed on my back in a huge rosebush and lay there wondering what had happened. I didn't know if I had tripped over something or if my cane had slipped, but it was a soft landing and I wasn't hurt.

Well, I don't have to worry about the steps, I thought, and I started to get up but my feet weren't touching anything. I couldn't get any traction. I tried sitting up, but my coat was caught on something. I rolled to the left and a brier pricked my cheek. There was a large branch next to my face. If I rolled the other way, I'd be rolling into the bush.

Maybe I could break the branch next to my face, I thought. I pulled my coat sleeves down over my hands to protect them from briers and got a firm grip on the branch. It didn't even bend, and then I remembered that pipes were made from brier. I wasn't going to be able to break that limb. I was stuck. I couldn't get out. Welcome to the real world, I thought, and I started laughing at the whole ridiculous situation.

I lay there laughing until I realized that I was going to be there all night and in the morning the rock would come out of the house and find me. I had to get out of this bush.

Weight! If I was heavy enough the bush would bend and I

239

could get a foot on the ground. I unbuttoned my raincoat except for the last button, spread it open like a bowl, and waited for it to collect rain.

My arms, dangling at my side, began to ache, so I folded them on my chest and waited . . . and waited . . . and waited until I could stand the boredom no longer. I explored the pockets of the coat and found a cigar and two books of matches. My father must have worn my coat at some time.

I wondered if I could get a cigar lit in the rain. I stuck the cigar in my mouth and struck a match. It went out. A second. It went out. I tried striking two at a time, and then three. the first book of matches ran out and I hadn't come close to getting the cigar lit. I struck the entire second book against the empty jacket of the first and puffed wildly on the cigar— and it fired to life. I folded my hands on my chest and puffed on the cigar and waited.

The cigar was more than half gone when the headlights hit me. The family! Jesus. What would they think? They'll think I'm drunk. They'll think there's a drunk lying in their rosebush. I hope her old man ain't the violent type, I thought.

A man and woman got out of the car and approached cautiously, stopping several feet away. They looked at me and then at each other.

"Are you all right?" the man asked.

I took the cigar out of my mouth and said, "I don't seem to be able to get out of this bush."

"How'd you get in there?" he asked, not moving forward or offering to help. The woman stepped closer to him.

"I fell off the porch."

"He's not drunk, is he, George?" the woman whispered.

"I don't know. I don't think so," he told her. "You say you fell off the porch?"

"My cane slipped, I think. It should be lying around here somewhere," I told him. "Anyway, I fell off the porch."

"Oh, my God," the woman moaned when she saw the cane.

240

"Help him, George. Don't just stand there. Are you hurt?"

"No, I'm just stuck."

He offered a hand, I clasped it and was pulled from the thorny embrace of the rosebush. When I stood up I felt mud ooze over my right foot and for the first time I realized I had lost a shoe.

"Come on in the house and let's get you dried off," she said.

I thought of the girl somewhere in the house and the embarrassment was too much. "I think I'll just grab a hot shower when I get home," I told her.

The man handed me my shoe and the woman said, "How long have you been out here?"

"Not long," I said. "About an hour."

"Good Lord. Why didn't you call Gloria?"

I didn't know what to say to that so I said, "I did call her. I guess she just didn't hear me."

From the look on the woman's face I knew Gloria was going to catch hell and that pleased me. I'm not sure why, but it somehow seemed just.

When I got home it was still early and everybody was still up. I sat in the car for a while, dreading going in looking the way I did. There were scratches all over my face, my hair was plastered to my head, one foot was muddy halfway to my knee, I was soaked, and I hadn't been able to get my shoe back on.

I put it off as long as I could. Finally I walked up to the door, opened it, and stood there with my shoe in my hand.

A look of horror flashed across my mother's face and she gasped. She didn't say anything, she just looked at me. Then she turned to Wayne and said, "Just what kind of girl was that?"

21

"BUT we have no assurance that you can pull an eight-hour day. It's been a long time since you've worked and, considering the physical changes that have taken place . . . well . . ." He let the words hang there and shook his head.

"An eight-hour day would be coasting for me, Mr. Waddell. For the past few years my workday has been a lot longer than eight hours."

"I'm sure that's true, but we're talking about a different situation altogether."

"I realize that, but I don't feel that the physical demands of this job will prove to be any more—"

"I think I'm in a better position to make a judgment as to the demands of this job than you are," he said, and his voice was sharp and cutting.

Was I being argumentative? Maybe so, but he was slipping away and I couldn't continue to let that happen.

"Let me ask you something, Mr. Waddell. Do you care how your employees get to work? I mean, does it matter whether they come by bus, or drive a new car, or an old car, or ride a bike? Does it make any difference?"

242

"Well, of course not. As long as they get here on time and do their job, it's of no concern to me how they get here."

"Then why should the vehicle they use once they get in the building make any difference? As long as they do their job."

"The vehicle they use once they're in the building?" he said with a frown.

"Their bodies, Mr. Waddell. Simple vehicles, nothing more. You wouldn't care if I drove to work in a battered wreck, you've already said so. So why should it make any difference how I get around the office, as long as I do the job?"

"I see. That's an interesting idea, one I'd never thought of," he said. "But that still leaves us with the fact that I don't feel you can handle the physical demands of this particular job."

"Look, Mr. Waddell"—desperation burned at the edges of my voice—"I'll work free. I'll work for one month, and if at the end of that time I'm not doing the job better than anybody ever has, you just tell me and that'll be the end of it. If I am doing it, then put me on the payroll."

"Now you're getting into violation of federal wage and hour laws and God knows what else. No, I'm afraid we can't allow you to work without pay, but I'll tell you what I can do—there's a meeting of personnel directors this Thursday night. I'll be glad to take your application to the meeting and see if anyone has an opening that you can fill."

I tried to prevent it, but I could feel the lines tighten at the corners of my mouth and eyes. I could feel the blood begin to pound at my temples. I wanted to unload all the frustration of the past six months, frustration that was building into rage. But I could not do that because Waddell had not slammed the door, and if I unleashed my anger the door would close and with it the possibility that someone at that meeting would have something.

No one ever slammed the door. There was always the promise, the possibility, a phone call, a man to see, an idea to be

243

taken up with superiors. They were interested, concerned, shocked that six months of effort had not produced a job of any kind. And their admiration, their sympathy, their embarrassment were always followed by the standard form letter thanking me for my interest and expressing regret that there was nothing for me at this time.

"If you'll do that I'll appreciate it," I said, standing to leave. "And I appreciate your taking the time to see me."

"It was my pleasure. I think you're a remarkable young man, Mr. Helms, and I'm sure that with your tenacity it will be just a matter of time before something breaks for you. Thanks for considering us."

I dragged my left foot as I walked across the lobby to the elevator, and the sound disgusted me. My walking always seemed to be worse after an interview, or maybe I was just more sensitive to it. Interviews left me depressed, with a feeling of worthlessness, and the shuffling sound of a dragging foot only enhanced the feeling.

The receptionist was standing up and bending over her desk for something when I walked across the lobby. Her skirt rose up in the back, revealing long, smooth legs and the lacy edge of white panties. It had been a lifetime since I had touched the silky skin of a woman's thigh or felt the inviting warmth of flesh beneath the thin fabric of feminine attire.

I had noticed her while I was waiting for the interview. I had watched her move around the lobby with a fluid grace that was maddening. I had noticed the gentle sway of her full breasts, the way her skirt clung to the curve of her buttocks as she moved in long, graceful strides across the lobby. I had watched the shape of her legs change as she knelt to pick up a dropped pencil and the imprint of her bra straining against her blouse when she reached behind her for an envelope. I had watched, and as I did I remembered other days and other women, and an ancient need grew in me.

I glanced at my watch. It was a few minutes before twelve

244

and I decided to give it a try. Anything was better than going home and staring at the phone, trying to think of someone to call, or leafing through that hopelessly out-of-date address book on the chance that I had overlooked someone the last time.

"Do you go to lunch at twelve?" I asked, stepping up to the desk.

"Yes, I do," she said with a smile.

"Well, I know it's not the most original approach in the world, but you've got to eat and I've got to eat, and I know it would be a lot more enjoyable for me if we did it together. So, if you haven't made other plans, I'd like to buy you lunch."

"Why, thank you. That's very thoughtful of you, but I'm afraid I've already made plans. It was very nice of you to ask, though."

"Maybe some other time," I said, turning to leave.

I wished I could turn faster. It always made me feel foolish to have to stand there so long after I had been turned down. It was one thing to be able to walk away, but it was embarrassing to have to stand there and slowly turn. I didn't know whether to grin or what, and I always got the feeling that the girl seeing me struggle to turn was glad she had said no.

And who could blame her for saying no, I thought as I finally walked away from the desk. That was a crude approach. She was a good-looking girl and used to guys asking. With a girl like that I should have come up with something besides "You've got to eat—I've got to eat." But she did seem sincere, and it wasn't her fault that she had already made plans. She even seemed pleased that I asked and that was a good feeling—a damn good feeling.

Just as I reached the elevator a girl stuck her head in and yelled, "Hey, Susan, we're going down to Rico's for a sandwich. You wanta go?"

I looked back over my shoulder just as the receptionist said, "Yes, wait a minute. Let me get my purse."

I bit my lip hard and my face reddened with anger. Anger for the girl at first, but then for myself for putting myself in that position. I never should have asked—not for the reasons I did, not out of need. I wished doggedly that I had been strong enough not to give in to that need, but I wasn't, and there would be other times. I would ask again, and each time I was driven to it I would hate myself a little more. I was suddenly consumed with an overwhelming contempt for my body and for myself for being bound to it.

When I reached the car, I sat down and breathed easier. It was good to be off my unsteady legs and I was thankful for the long drive home. It always relaxed me and gave the anger time to subside. I did not want the eager, expectant faces that awaited me at home to see me like this.

I decided to take the back roads instead of the new interstate. It would take longer, but I needed the time and I enjoyed the slower pace of the country roads. I could feel the muscles of my shoulders beginning to relax and the deep, tense lines of my face beginning to smooth as I drove past the small farms that dotted the land. They were abandoned for the most part, having belonged to another more simple time, but cotton still grew wild in scattered bouquets across deserted fields and in small clusters nestled against ramshackle houses, and I couldn't help wondering if life wouldn't have been easier back then. I would have died back then, I told myself quickly, and the thought lost its fascination. I would have died in a ditch in Asheville because no one would have known what to do for a broken neck. I let the thought go and reached up and switched on the radio.

I knew something was wrong as soon as I walked in the house. My mother's expression spoke eloquently of tragedy.

"What's wrong?" I said, convinced that something had happened to my brother or my father.

"Maybe you better sit down," she said.

"What's happened?" I asked, slipping out of my coat.

246

"I ran into Mrs. Brockman today. It's Cindy Davis."

"What about her?" I asked with growing concern.

"She's dead, Tom," she said in a frail, childlike voice.

"Cindy? Not Cindy. Are you sure . . . did Mrs. Brockman—"

"I'm sure."

"How . . . what . . . a blood clot? What?"

"No." She looked down and the silence seemed bottomless. When she did look up her eyes were filled with tears. "She killed herself," she got out before her voice broke.

"No! Not Cindy! Cindy wouldn't . . ." I bit my trembling lip hard, walked across the room and slammed my fist into the back of a chair. "For God's sake, why? What could have driven her to that?"

"They don't know."

"Did she leave a note?"

"No, nothing."

"Well, what was going on? Had something happened?"

"They don't know."

"What do you mean, they don't know?" I flared up angrily. "Where was her family? Did anybody see any signs? Surely to God something must have happened."

"They just don't know, son. She finished school and seemed to be doing fine. She had been looking for a job for six or eight months—I'm not sure—Mrs. Brockman wasn't sure how long. Nothing unusual had happened. Her parents have gone over and over the past days and months, and absolutely nothing happened that would cause this."

"Well, something happened," I said bitterly.

I left the house early the next morning and spent the entire day going to employment agencies. It kept me from thinking. I hadn't slept much the night before—I kept thinking about Cindy and wondering. I was still wondering when I got home.

There was a car parked in the drive, so I parked in front of the house and cursed under my breath. I took my time

247

walking up the drive and paused, taking a deep breath before entering the house. I didn't want my mother to see the strain of the day that I knew was etched in my face.

"Well, it's about time. We'd just about given up on you," Rick said as I came into the house.

"Well, well. If it isn't the reluctant warrior," I said with a broad smile. "How go the wars?"

"Win a few, lose a few. But those are painful memories, son. Never ask an old warrior to recount his days of battle. Besides, I'm a civilian now."

"With only an occasional nightmare to remind you of your days of glory, huh?"

"That and the bloody malaria. The jungles of New Jersey were a living pesthole, full of loan sharks and whores, pimps and pushers." He shook his head remorsefully. "A man had to keep a constant vigil just to stay alive—but I survived and I'm a better man for it."

"A bigger one, too. How much do you weigh?"

"Ten pounds more than I should," he said, slapping his stomach. "But less than I'm going to. Don't take off your coat, I'm taking you to dinner."

"As long as you're paying," I told him. I looked at Mom and shook my head at the question her expression asked about the day's events.

"You two run on," she told us. "I know you've got things to talk about that no mother should ever hear."

Rick kissed her on the cheek and said, "It's good to see you again, Mom, and it's great to be home."

"When did you get out?" I asked as he backed out of the drive.

"About ten days ago. I just got in today, though," he explained. "I've been in Winston-Salem, looking for a job. I stopped off there on my way home."

"Any luck?"

"Yeah. I got on in the accounting department of Hanes."

"Accounting department? What do you know about accounting?"

"Nothing. Absolutely zilch. They're going to train me."

"Is there any reason I couldn't do that job? I mean, is there anything required that I couldn't handle physically?"

"Hell, no. It's a desk job. All I'll have to do is go to a filing cabinet or someone's desk once in a while."

"How about accounting? Did you have more than the two basic courses?"

"Nope. I had the same thing you did."

"Shit."

"Why?"

"I've been pounding the pavement for six months and I'm either overqualified or underqualified or there is some physical aspect of the job that they don't feel I can handle. And that's true in some cases. Some jobs require things I can't do, but ninety percent of the desk jobs don't require a damn thing more than yours."

"Six months," he said with disbelief. "Man, I had three interviews and I was suicidal. I got knee-walking, falling-down, passing-out drunk after each one and you can damn well bet I took the first offer I got. I hate those things. They take away your self-respect or your confidence or something. I came out of each one feeling . . . I don't know. Feeling like . . ."

"How do you think I feel?"

"That's different. You can handle it, I can't. It's like speech class—I went all to pieces just knowing I had to get up there and talk, but you breezed through, didn't even prepare, you made it up on the spot."

"Interviews aren't speech class, and I come out of them feeling just like you—like I've tried to sell my soul and there were no buyers, at any price. And the funny thing is, I go into each one dead sure I'm going to get it, not a doubt in the world. Man, they're going to be lucky to get me." I laughed bitterly. "That's a joke."

"Not me. I crawl in and whatever's lower than crawl is how I come out."

"How did you hear about Hanes?"

"Through an agency. They set up all my interviews. Have you tried an agency?"

"I've signed up with nine so far and not one interview. The only thing I got from them is a list of every employer in Charlotte that employs more than twenty people, and I'm working my way down that list."

"You're just going out cold?"

"What else can I do? I tried it by types of business at first. I hit all the banks, then all the insurance companies and so on, but then I said to hell with that and started on page one heading for God knows what."

"How about here at home?"

"Yep. I tried the banks, the insurance companies, the telephone company, the hospital, a few of those small hosiery mills and even those half-assed finance companies—nothing."

"Damn," he said. "You haven't gone to the mill, have you?"

I looked at him with astonishment.

"Good. There for a minute I thought . . ."

"No way. There's no way I'll ever go to the mill."

Later as we sat in the restaurant, he looked at me and smiled secretively.

"I want you to do something for me," he said.

"What?"

"Be in my wedding."

"You're kidding."

"Nope. I told you those interviews left me suicidal."

"Who's the unlucky girl?"

"The one I wrote you about, Barbara. Barbara Queen."

"Oh, yeah. But I didn't think it was that serious."

"It wasn't until it came time to pack up and pull out."

"Well? When and where?"

"Next month. The twenty-fifth, in Norwich, Connecticut."

"Connecticut? Are you crazy? I can't go to Connecticut."

"Why not?"

"I don't have any money. My folks give me gas money and lunch money every day, but I couldn't ask them . . . I mean, it's bad enough to ask them for that."

"Well, I sure as hell don't have any. How about Wayne?"

"He's in college. Did you have any money when you were in college?"

Rick shrugged.

"About all I can do is congratulate you," I said, reaching across the table shaking his hand. "That's also your wedding present."

"I wish you could be there," he said regretfully.

"Yeah, I do too."

"Ah, well." He shrugged. "It may be for the best. My old man is going to act as best man, which means you'd have to be an usher, and to tell you the truth, I think it would take you the better part of a week to fill up the church."

"At least a couple of days." I laughed. "But then, it all depends on what you're looking for—quantity or quality. I might not seat many of 'em, but it would be done with style and grace."

"With me waiting in the wings to go on a honeymoon? I don't care about style and grace—what I want is speed."

"I can't blame you for that."

"I want you to meet Barbara. I think you'll like her."

"Yeah, I'm looking forward to it."

"Your mom told me about Cory," he said, looking at me seriously. "I hated to hear that."

"Me too," I said with a smile of sad resignation. "But it didn't come as any big surprise."

"Are you dating anybody?"

"In Concord? Be serious. Who's to date in Concord?"

"There's bound to be somebody."

"Believe me, there's nobody. I've tried everything. There

are no clubs in this town and it's an off year politically, so there are no campaigns to join. I even went to a damn ceramics class at the rec center." I leaned forward. "I even went to church," I said confidentially.

"Church," he said with alarm. "You went to church?"

"Yeah," I answered suspiciously, surprised by his reaction. "What's wrong with that?"

"You went to church? To get laid?"

"I didn't go to get laid," I said indignantly.

"What did you go for?"

"To meet a girl."

"And what were you going to do if you met a girl?"

I grinned at him.

"You see! You went to get laid. Goddamn, you're gonna burn in hell."

"Probably. But if it'll make you feel any better, I planned to wait until after the service."

"Well, that's different." He laughed.

"It's still pretty bad," I said. "I wish there was a pill or something you could take because some days I'm flat climbing the walls. I mean, you go out every day and the streets are full of little secretaries and every office you go in has a receptionist sitting there with her skirt hiked up to her navel or wearing something braless, and then you come home all fired up and there's not a damn thing to do. There's not even anybody to call, so you sit around feeling mean as hell, hating everybody, but most of all hating yourself for having the need."

"You haven't had a date since before you went in the hospital?"

I held up a single finger.

"One date," he exclaimed. "One lousy date in four years?"

"Lousy isn't exactly the word I'd use. That night has to go down as one of the all-time bad nights of my life—pure disaster."

"Son, that's a broad statement, 'cause we've had some bad nights."

"Believe me, it's a winner," I insisted. "Wayne fixed me up with the older sister of some girl he was dating, and I'm going to have to be a lot drunker than I am now to tell you about it. But you won't have to wait long. When we leave here we'll go hoist a few to celebrate your last few days as a free man. Let's really tie one on."

"I always said you were destined to make great decisions and this should rank among the top. Tonight may well go down as our finest hour."

"No. Our finest hour came with the redheaded twins."

"True," Rick agreed. "I'd almost forgotten that—God knows I've tried."

"And well you should," I said, looking beyond him. With an expression of interior pain I quickly dropped my glance.

Rick turned and looked over his shoulder just as the girl averted her eyes. He looked questioningly at me and said, "What's wrong with that?" jerking his thumb in the direction of the girl.

"Nothing, but it's not what it seems."

"Don't tell me," he argued. "I know that look."

"I can't play the game by the old rules anymore, not even the little eye games. When I picked up this cane all the rules changed."

He shook his head in disgust.

"Okay, I'll explain. You're right about the look, it means what it's always meant, but the key in this case is who came in first, and I came in first so it doesn't mean anything."

"Who came in first? Who gives a damn who came in first? She's interested and that's that."

"If she had come in first that's what it would mean, but she didn't so it doesn't," I said with a grin.

"I feel a drunk coming on," he moaned. "You don't make sense."

"If she had gotten here first, she would have seen us walk in, right?"

"Right."

"If she had seen us walk in and still looked at me like that, it would mean what it used to and I could take it from there. But she didn't see me walk. She doesn't know about the cane and she's gonna be embarrassed when we get up to leave."

"Why embarrassed?"

"What's she doing? She's staring at me, right? Flirting but staring, right?"

"Yeah."

"That's an unpardonable sin—staring at a cripple."

"But she doesn't know you're crippled," he protested.

"It doesn't matter. She'll think that I thought that's why she was looking, and she'll feel awful about it."

"Why will she think that?"

"I don't know," I confessed. "I guess that when I stand up she'll see how I walk and she'll wish she had known that, because if she had she wouldn't have been interested and she wouldn't have looked. Now, she knows that I knew it all the time, and therefore I knew she couldn't be interested so she must have been staring out of curiosity."

He stared at me with a vacant expression. "Huh?"

"Look, it's like the girls in the lounges. They will assume that I think that the only possible reason they would stare is out of curiosity. They will assume that I have sense enough to realize that they're not going to find me physically attractive."

"How do you know that?"

"I know because of the expression on her face when we get up to leave. I know because the only girls that flirt with me are the ones that come in after I do, and the ones in the car beside me at the stop light, and the ones that haven't seen me walk."

"Let's go."

"Now?"

"I want to see her face."

"Well, wait a minute."

"Come on, she might leave," he said, standing and reaching for his wallet to leave a tip.

I stood up and pulled the cane out from under the table. As we walked by the girl she glanced up with an uncertain smile and an expression that said I'm sorry, I didn't know.

When we stopped at the cashier's booth, Rick looked back toward the girl and then at me. "That's the first time I ever saw anybody apologize with their face."

I grinned triumphantly at him.

"There ain't nothing simple anymore, is there?"

I thought about Cindy and said, "No, there isn't anything simple—not anymore."

22

I wasn't looking forward to seeing Willard Wilks, and I didn't want to go to vocational rehab. It was Willard who had pushed Dr. Walters into discharging me from the hospital. I used to hate his visits. I felt like a trained animal showing him what I could do that I hadn't been able to do on his prior visit. He was never pleased with my progress, so I stopped trying to show him anything. I referred him to Stirewalt or told him to check the chart, and he had come to dislike me as much as I did him.

I hated the idea of asking him for help, but it was an avenue I hadn't explored, maybe the only one. More than a year had slipped away from me since I went on that first interview and if I had known then how hard it was going to be to find a job, I wouldn't have been so relieved when they told me it had been filled. I would have found a way of crossing that street.

I walked into the building and found the office I was looking for.

"I'd like to see Willard Wilks, please."

"Mr. Wilks is no longer with us. Mr. William France has taken over his caseload."

"Could I talk to him then?"

"Do you have an appointment?"

I looked at the woman and wondered if she was retarded. She had no physical signs of a handicap, but she was working for VR, so maybe hers was mental.

"No, ma'am." I smiled. "I didn't even know he existed until just now."

"Well, have a seat," she said without smiling. "He'll see you when he can. What's your name? Do we have a file on you?"

"Tom Helms, and yes, I think you have my file."

I sat down and waited and wondered why everything to do with the handicapped was second class. I looked at the dirty, chipped, brown tile floors and the scarred walls and thought of the plush, carpeted offices I had seen. The office furniture looked as though it had been salvaged from some disaster and, judging from Willard, the people had been reclaimed from some human garbage dump. I felt out of place and ill at ease. I was about to leave when a young man walked in looking as out of place as I felt.

"Mr. Helms? I'm Bill France. Let's go into my office."

The office was a shambles. There was no room on the desk to do more than lay his file. It was covered with stacks of folders. Several of the drawers of the battered filing cabinet were so overstuffed they refused to close.

"I was looking over your file. It's been a while—but you've come a long way. Willard had written you off a little too soon." He laughed. "But Willard had a habit of doing that. I think he wrote himself off somewhere around the age of three."

"He wasn't one of my favorite people." I smiled, and I immediately liked Bill France.

"Well, Tom, what can I do for you?"

"I was hoping you could help me find a job."

Bill frowned. "Okay." He nodded. "First let me explain something. We're set up to vocationally rehabilitate those that need it. That's our primary function—to provide whatever services, whatever training, whatever education it takes to make an individual vocationally independent. Now, you have your degree, you have an education—the tools, if you will—and you are physically capable of using those tools, so you have no need of the services I'm set up to provide. That degree, in this particular situation, in regard to what I can do for you, is going to be a handicap."

My brow furrowed.

"Would you like to learn watch repair?"

I shook my head. "I don't think so."

"But if you didn't have that degree you might. If you didn't have that degree you might be happy to go into any number of trade schools I could get you in. I just want you to understand the situation I'm in, what I can do and what I can't do. Hell, if you didn't have that degree we could send you to school to get it. In fact, we have a masters program—would you be interested in going back and picking up a masters?"

"If I have to. I don't want to go back to school, but if it's the only way I can get a job, I'll go."

"How long have you been looking?"

"Over a year."

"Jesus Christ," he moaned. "Before I took this job I wouldn't have believed that, I just would not have believed it, but now it doesn't even surprise me anymore. I'll do what I can, but about all I can do is make a few calls; there are some companies we've had success dealing with and a few others I might be able to make see the light. But what have you done, where have you been? There's no need to cover the same ground."

I took the list with its battered, frayed pages out of my coat pocket and tossed it on the desk.

"The ones with the check marks are the ones I've seen. Double checks beside the ones I've seen twice. Besides that, I'm signed up with thirteen personnel agencies—they haven't come up with a single interview. I've taken the Federal Civil Service exam and the state merit exam, and I watch the want ads. I've called the Governor's Committee on Employment of the Handicapped and was told that their function was to make the public aware of the need to employ the handicapped—not to assist individuals in finding employment. I've written to the state representative from my district and to my senator in Washington—nothing. I even called that reporter on the *Observer* and tried to get him to do a story on me. You know the one that's always doing those human interest stories—and then he does a follow-up on how much better their life became after the story. He said it was a story too often told and he had written it too many times."

"Damned if you ain't 'bout touched all the bases," he said. Then he took out a pen and wrote a name and address on a card. "Do you know where the Dixie Motel is out at Twenty-nine?"

"Yeah, I think so."

"Well, get in touch with Mr. Bostic, give him this card and tell him I sent you. If that doesn't work out, let me know and I'll make a few calls."

I thanked him and left with the feeling that together we might be able to accomplish what I had not been able to do alone.

Forty-five minutes later I sat in the office of the Dixie Motel talking with Fred Bostic.

"As I explained to Mr. France, this is a night clerk's job—eleven to seven. It doesn't require much. Can you run a switchboard?"

"Yes," I lied.

"Well, the pay ain't much, not for somebody that's been to college," he said, more to himself than to me, as he lit a cigar. He studied the glowing end of his cigar for a minute and then said, "I don't think it'll work. There are times when people come in here with babies, and you'd have to carry a crib upstairs for them. I just don't think you'd be able to manage that."

"I can handle it. I'll get the crib up there if I have to strap it to my back."

259

"And then," Bostic said thoughtfully, "there are other things that come up from time to time."

"I can do the job, Mr. Bostic. I know I can. Just let me try. If it doesn't work out, you can always let me go. But at least give me a shot at it," I said, and the anguish in my voice made me sick to my stomach. Had I been reduced to this? Begging for a night clerk's job in a motel? And what if I got it, where would it lead, to a day clerk's job? Bostic was the day clerk. This wasn't a chain. It was a one-man operation. I was begging for a dead-end job in a flea-bag motel. I wondered what Cory would think of me now. God, what if she and her doctor checked in one night.

"No. I think we'd better forget it this time, but I'll keep your name and number, and if anything else comes up I'll let you know."

I almost laughed, partly from relief and partly because the statement was so typical and so ludicrous—what would possibly come up? There were no other jobs in the place, nothing.

In the weeks that followed, Bill sent me on three more interviews. I got the feeling that they were seeing me because Bill refused to take no for an answer and the only way to get him off their backs was at least to go through the motions of an interview.

"You can't honestly tell me that it's the height of your ambition to be an account clerk," Mr. Edwards was saying.

"If I did you'd know I was lying, wouldn't you?" I asked with a smile.

He smiled back. "Damn right I would. And you'll leave the minute you find something better. Now don't tell me you won't."

"Normally, yes, I would. But I need to establish a recent work history. I need to prove a few things to those people that have the better jobs. What if I agreed to stay with you for at least two years?"

He shook his head.

"What have you got to lose? You can fire me if I'm not doing the job, and if I am, you know you've got a good employee for at least two years."

"Well, that may be true," he said, fidgeting with the application. "I didn't want to mention this, but we're going to run into a problem with insurance regulations. You see, the present policy we're under prohibits the employment of anyone with a handicap; our policy would have to be rewritten and our rates would skyrocket. In fact, it would cost us more in increased premiums than we have budgeted for this position."

I was stunned. I felt like I had been slapped in the face. It was a lie. It was one of the oldest dodges there was. I thought those days were over. I had believed them and their promises and they were all lying. They were all hiding and that's what Cindy must have realized. Jesus Christ!

The man didn't want me. None of them wanted me. I could do the job. I was overqualified. I had said I would stay—I wouldn't leave even if something better came along. He didn't want me for one reason—I was crippled. That's what Cindy had finally realized.

"If that's the case, I don't see any need to take any more of your time," I said, standing up and walking out of the office.

"You realize my hands are tied in this matter," he shouted after me.

When I reached the street I took in a deep breath of fresh air and held it, then I let it out slowly. I felt like a fool. I had believed all their lies. I had believed them. I hadn't believed Bo, and he had been closer to the truth than either of us realized. Why bust your ass? he asked. To be able to punch a button with your chin? It ain't worth the effort, he had said, and he was right. That's what Cindy had finally come to realize. It wasn't worth the effort. The only job I would ever get— the only job they would ever let me have—would be one that was of no more value to me than pushing that button had been to Bo. Pushing that button wouldn't have changed his life. It wouldn't have gotten him out of that bed. It wouldn't have brought anything he needed into his miserable life.

And that was what I had been killing myself for—to push a lousy button. I had been going out day after day, month after month, begging, pleading, smiling, bowing and scraping, and for what? Some menial job that would not allow me to have one single thing I had stayed alive for, that would not bring anything I needed into my life. I was on the garbage heap and didn't have the brains to realize it. I'd been thrown away and just didn't know it. Well, I knew it now. Bo was right. Cindy was right. The only place left for me wasn't worth the effort to get there.

I walked down to my car and sat there for a long time. I wasn't going on any more interviews. I wasn't going to listen to any more lies. I wasn't sure what I was going to do, but I wasn't going to do that and I wasn't going to go home.

I pulled the car into traffic and headed across town.

I heard Stirewalt's voice before I reached the gym.

"Dammit, Miss May, you're gonna get outta that chair if I have to pull you out of it."

I stood at the door and watched.

"Do you want your grandchildren to know what a pain in the ass you've been? Don't you want them to be proud of you? Dammit, listen to me, look up here."

I guessed the woman who was ignoring Stirewalt to be in her eighties, and judging from the short leg brace and the arm sling I knew she must have had a stroke. I had never understood why, but the older patients enjoyed Stirewalt's rough language, even those that chastised him for its use. Maybe it was because everyone else was so careful around them.

Stirewalt reached for the canvas sash around her waist and she began to yell.

"Don't start that! It won't do you a damn bit of good."

"Why don't you pick on somebody your own size, foul mouth," I said slowly and evenly.

Stirewalt turned around and broke into a slow smile when he saw me.

"Well, well, well, if it ain't the hard nose."

"You down to picking on old ladies?" I said without smiling.

"It helps keep my mean mean." He smiled. "But look at you. By God, you did it, didn't you?"

"I thought I told you I'd do it," I said with a puzzled look. "Didn't I mention something about that before I left?"

"Seems to me it did come up, but let's see you move. For all I know somebody might have carried you in here and propped you against that door."

Stirewalt watched me with a practiced eye as I made my way across the gym. Whistling through his teeth, he shook his head and said, "That's without a doubt the worst walking pattern I've ever seen."

"The key word in that sentence is *walking*. It is a pattern and it is walking."

"I thought you were going down with every step."

"You see any braces? You see any wheels? A minute ago I was over there, now I'm over here, and it just cost you one cup of coffee."

"Win a few, lose a few," he said, wrapping a big arm around my shoulders. "One cup of coffee coming up." Stirewalt caught an aide's eye and nodded toward Miss May, then he slowed his pace and moved behind me, watching my left foot as we walked down the hall. "Ever consider bracing that left foot?" he asked, moving up beside me.

"I've thought about it, but it won't work."

"Why not?"

"A spring-loaded brace will trigger the spasticity. Any pressure on the ball of my foot will trigger it. A brace would keep constant pressure on it, and the spasms won't ever stop."

"What about locking the ankle? That would keep the toe up."

"And what happens when the spasticity pulls the toe down? My foot's gonna come out of my shoe or my knee is going to

263

buckle—either way something's got to give."

When we reached the lounge, Stirewalt pulled a chair away from a table and motioned for me to sit down; then he knelt on one knee and picked up my left foot. He jammed the heel of his hand against the ball of the foot and immediately set off a series of spasms that continued until he eased his hand away.

"I didn't think they were that strong," he said, standing up and walking over to the coffee machine. When he returned he set a cup in front of me and said, "Try to brace that foot and you've got problems."

"Why is it that every time I tell you something you repeat it five minutes later and act like it's a brand-new idea?"

"Maybe I'm slow," he said. "But not as slow as some people I know. It's been three years and not a word from you."

"It's been over three and I didn't have anything to say."

"You never change, do you?"

"No."

"I was telling someone about you yesterday. We've got an eighteen-year-old quad—his brother was cleaning a gun and it went off. I'd like for him to see you."

"I'd rather not."

"It won't take but a minute."

I shook my head.

"What the hell's wrong with you? I just want you to talk to the kid."

"And tell him what? That if he busts his guts it's worth it?"

"Yeah, is that asking too much?"

"I don't believe it anymore, and I'm not going back there and lie to him, and I'm sure as hell not going to tell him the truth."

"You don't think it's worth it? You don't think that what you have now is better than what you had then?"

"We're not talking about me, we're talking about him. You want me to tell him that if he busts his ass and if he can survive

264

then there's some kind of decent life waiting for him, and that just ain't true."

"Who the hell are you to make that kind of decision?"

"What do you think I've been doing for the last year and a half?" I flared up angrily. "Chasing that rainbow, and there ain't no pot of gold. Do you remember Cindy Davis, huh? You remember her? You called her a champion once, remember?"

"Yes."

"Well, after fighting her way out of here and after fighting her way through college and after nine months of looking for a job—looking for some kind of decent life—she sat in her bedroom and took those fancy braces you made for her hands and opened a vein and quietly bled to death."

"Oh my God," Stirewalt moaned.

"I wasn't sure why, not then. It was too soon. But I know now. It wasn't any great trauma, no single crushing blow. It was a gentle, slow washing away of all her pride and courage and self-respect. It took more courage for her to leave the safety of her house each day than the average son-of-a-bitch will ever be able to dredge up. And then she spent that day— every day—listening to the same son-of-a-bitch tell her what she couldn't do, why she wouldn't fit in. She spent the day being written off by people who would have folded a hundred times if they had had to go through what she had. Then one day she began to believe them, she began to see herself as they saw her—and one day there wasn't any more courage, there wasn't any more hope. It just happened one day—a day no different from all the others. The courage simply ran out."

Stirewalt stared at the table and ran a finger absently through loose grains of sugar collected in a small pile, and silence hung in the air like the aftermath of a scream.

"And she was a champion," I said softly. "Is that kid you want me to talk to a champion? Is Matthew Sims a champion? Or Althea Biggers?"

265

He didn't answer me. He sat staring at the table. When he looked up, his eyes were filled with pain and his face held a weariness I had not seen before.

"I don't know," he said quietly, almost in a whisper. "I just don't know. You work and you . . . and then you send them . . ." He looked back down at the table and shook his head sadly. "You say you've been at it for a year and a half?" he asked, glancing up at me.

I nodded.

"If you don't believe it's worth it, how can you do it?"

"I don't have the courage Cindy had. I'm not as brave as she was. But I don't need courage, not as long as I can get mad—and they manage to make me mad every day."

"And every day it costs you something."

"It didn't at first. At first I was just knocking on doors that wouldn't open, but now I leave a little piece of myself behind. I'm losing something. I don't know exactly what, but something's dying."

"The same thing that died in Cindy?"

"I don't know. But sometimes I want to stand in the street and scream for help. Sometimes I just want to scream 'Help me, for God's sake, won't somebody help me.' And sometimes I get so scared I start shaking. Sometimes I sit in the car and sweat like a whore trying to get up the courage to cross another street or climb another flight of steps. And the only way I can do it is to get mad at myself for being scared."

"I wish there was something—"

"There isn't. I shouldn't have flared up like that. It's just been a bad day," I told him. "What happend to Althea?"

"I don't know," he said, and we talked for a while until he looked at his watch and said, "I've got a meeting. Why don't you stick around and we'll have lunch."

"You gotta be out of your head. Eat this food when I don't have to? No way."

"Well, come on, I'll walk you out."

When we reached the door he said, "If I didn't have this meeting."

"Don't worry about it. It's a workday for you. We can socialize some other time."

"You'll come back, then?"

"Yeah, sure."

"Make it sometime soon, okay?"

"You got it," I told him, and we both knew I wouldn't be back.

23

I STOOD in the door and watched the postman make his way up the walk. Rain fell in sheets, pushed one way and then another by a whimsical wind. It danced across the walk and splashed under his feet and turned his pants black below the knees.

The wind swept across the door and its chill sent a shudder through me. Another summer had come and gone. Another year had slipped away. And the aching press of lost time weighed more heavily upon me each day. People had died and others had been born. They got married and they got divorced. Girls once too young to date were getting married, and neighborhood children were going off to college or joining the army or the Peace Corps. That great rush of life flowed like a swift river, it flowed around me and by me and was leaving me behind.

"Nasty day, huh?" the postman said, handing me the mail.

"Yes," I said, noticing two letters in company envelopes. Rejection letters. But the third was personal. It was small and addressed by hand.

I walked back to my room and tossed the two large envelopes on the desk and opened the small one. I unfolded the stationery and stared at it in mute shock. It was a birth announcement. Rick had a son. My God. Yesterday we were children, yesterday it was a game. Yesterday it was all ahead of me, and now it wasn't a game and more and more of life was behind me. It was slipping away in great chunks. Rick was a father. Rick had a job. Rick had a wife. Rick had a son. Rick had a life. Desperation screamed in my blood, it raged through my brain like fire before a strong wind. I was trapped. God, I was trapped and life was passing me by. I wanted to run into the street screaming. I had to get out. I had to change something.

I fought back the rising panic and picked up the phone. Shaking fingers fumbled over the dial.

"Let me speak to Bill France."

"Would you hold please."

I nervously worked the fingers of my right hand against the wood of the cane, not knowing what to do or where to go, but knowing I had to do something. I could not wait for this to pass as I had waited for so many other emotions to slowly die.

"Bill France."

"Bill, this is Tom. Have you got anything? Anything at all?"

"Yeah, I think so. Why don't you try a Mr. Pollard, he's in the American Building. There's a parking lot in the same block."

"Okay. Thanks."

"Wait a minute. Don't you want to know what he does?"

"What's he do?" I said, without interest.

"He runs a small chemical company. His offices are located in the American Building but his plant is out on Forty-nine. Ramco Chemical. Ever heard of them?"

"No."

"Listen, are you okay? You don't sound like yourself."

"I'm fine."

"Why don't you stop by here? We can have a cup of coffee and kick it around."

"I don't think so. Not today."

"Are you sure you're all right?"

"Yeah, I'm fine. Top of the world. Thanks, Bill. Thanks for everything."

I picked up a coat and tie and walked out of the house. I'd forgotten about the rain. I started back for a raincoat but that would take time and I was out of time.

Forty minutes later I sat in the office of Ramco Chemical, talking to Jay Pollard. I answered the first few questions automatically, without hearing what I said. I felt numb. Rick was a father. We were going to watch our children grow up together. We were going to sit around a grill on summer evenings, drinking Jack Daniels and remembering our boyhood and wondering if our sons were raising as much hell as we had. Panic kept jumping up and I kept fighting it back down.

"It's like I told France, I tried some of you people and the results haven't been very good."

I resented the term "you people." It stung and for a moment the fog lifted.

"What do you mean, 'you people'?"

"I mean you—you handicapped people," he said with a backward wave of his hand.

"Well, we handicapped people are carved from the mainstream of life. We weren't born into a race, or ordained into a sect, or recruited by any movement. We're just people—not *you* people—just people," I told him, but it lacked conviction. My voice did not have the cutting edge it should have had.

"Now, that's just what I'm talking about," he said angrily, pointing a stern finger at me. "You're bitter. You come in here with a chip on your shoulder, thinking the world owes you something."

"I haven't asked you for anything," I said softly. "I came here to sell you my abilities. And if not to sell, then to trade. To trade you a day's work for a day's pay."

"And you came in here hostile, challenging the first thing I said. I told France that I didn't want to see any more of you people. You're just like the last guy I hired that was crippled—you're touchy. A person never knows what to say around you. One wrong word, and you'll have the office in a turmoil all day. Well, I made that mistake once but I'm not about to make it again, no sir. I just don't think there's any place for you in my company."

"And what about your world," I breathed through clenched teeth, fighting back the scream that was rising in me.

"What? What was that?"

"Nothing," I said, standing up and walking out without looking up from the floor. I had to hold pack the panic. I had to think. For God's sake, won't somebody help me! The words echoed through me and I wanted to scream them at someone.

Where was the anger, I wondered as I stood on the street. Why wasn't I mad? Jesus, Rick had a son. He was leaving me behind. They were all leaving me behind. I had to do something.

I started up the street, stopped, turned around and started down the street. I had to go somewhere. Anywhere. But where?

I reached into my coat pocket and took out the worn, yellowed list of companies. I unfolded it and stood looking at names with double checks and triple checks by them as the rain splattered in dark spots against the paper. Until the ink began to run and the paper sagged limply in my hand. And then I knew where I would go. I let the sheet fall from my hand and flutter to the pavement.

I drove without thinking, without feeling. I drove out of Charlotte.

When I pulled into the parking lot, a guard motioned me toward a parking space.

"You going to personnel?"

"Yes," I said, stepping out of the car.

It stood there like a prison, that great red-brick building, and I stood looking at it, waiting, hoping the anger would come and I could turn and walk away. But the anger did not come and I could not walk away. I felt nothing. I walked across the parking lot toward the mill. And I felt nothing. I was going to work, and if the mill was all that was left, then I would have to accept that. The panic had passed and in its wake a cold resolve had risen. A resolve to survive. I would do what I had to do and if emotion came, if self-contempt arose, if pride died, then that was the price I would pay.

"I'd like to see somebody about a job," I told the receptionist.

"Do you have an appointment?"

"No, I'm sorry, I don't."

"Well, you'll want to see Mr. Holding. Would you fill out an application, please. He'll be with you in a moment."

I completed the application and returned it to the receptionist, and as I crossed the tile floor of the waiting room I noticed my cane slipping. When I sat down I looked at the rubber tip and was surprised to find it covered with cotton lint. There was no evidence of it on the floor, but one trip across that floor and my cane was covered with it. I cleaned the lint off and rolled it into a ball between my fingers, thinking of the games Rick and I had played with the lintheads; soon I would join their ranks, an office worker, but no different from those locked forever to the rattling looms.

I pressed the ball of lint between my fingers and wondered how many of them had died because their lungs were full of the stuff. I remembered watching my grandfather choke to death, and an old hatred stirred sluggishly.

"Mr. Helms, Mr. Holding will see you now."

"I was just looking over your application," Holding said, standing and extending his hand. He motioned for me to sit down.

"I see you went to Georgia. Why Georgia?"

"Because it's on a quarter system, and I was going to a school on the quarter system. I could transfer more credits."

"I see. I see," he said thoughtfully. "Why is it that you're twenty-eight years old and still single?" he asked, looking up at me with one eyebrow arched accusingly, a slow smile crawling across his mouth, curling it into a knowing sneer.

The implication was plain and the cocked eyebrow served only to enforce it. They even wanted to take that away from me, to question my manhood. It was just what I expected the mill to do, to strip you naked, to steal from you the last vestige of pride.

"If you'll notice, I went to college for four years, was in the hospital for two, convalesced for two, and I've been looking for a job for two years. That adds up to ten years, and I haven't been in a position to be able to afford to get married during that time."

"Oh," he said disappointedly, looking back at the application.

I wondered if he would have been happier if I had suddenly confessed to being homosexual.

"Well, exactly what type of work are you interested in, what do you think you'd like to do?"

"I realize it's not the best form to say anything, but that's exactly what I'm looking for—anything. I'll take absolutely anything I can get. I just want a job. I don't care what it is."

"Well, it would have to be something in the office, and unfortunately we don't have any openings at this time. There may be something coming up in accounts receivable in the near future. If you'd like, I'll keep your application on file."

I was stunned. I couldn't believe what I was hearing. The mill had always been there—reaching out, pulling the men off their farms, the women out of their homes, the children from their classrooms. I had spent a lifetime trying to escape its smothering embrace and now . . .

"Look, Mr. Holding"—desperation burned out the shame

in my face—"there must be something—anything. You've got fifteen thousand people working here. There must be something I can do."

"But only a small percentage of those are office personnel, and as I said, we don't have anything at this time," he said. "I'm afraid I'm going to have to cut this short, I'm due in a meeting. We'll keep your application on file. Thank you for coming by," he said, opening the door and standing by it.

I sat there in silence, staring at the floor, not knowing what to do or where to go. I had been willing—against all I believed—to come here. And now to find that there was no place for me, no need for me, not even here. I longed for the anger, waited for the purifying anger that would cleanse me of this unforgivable transgression, but the anger did not come.

I stood up and walked out without saying anything, without feeling anything—except an overwhelming shame.

I did not look up as I made my way down the hall, nor did I hear the hated rasping sound of my dragging foot. I pressed the button for the elevator and waited—waited for the anger to come. I stood quietly and waited for the veins at my temples to stand up and beat with my blood, waited for the sound of my heart to crowd out all hearing, waited for the searing rage to rise within me as it had always risen.

The elevator doors opened and still I waited. But the blood did not rise, my heart did not pound out its fury, nor did anything within me fan into flame. I stepped slowly onto the elevator and suddenly I knew: There would be no more anger.

I made my way out of the building and onto the busy street. Someone hurrying by bumped my shoulder, knocking me off balance. I staggered forward, wedging a shoulder against the building to keep from falling. I hung there for a moment, motionless, not feeling, not thinking. I turned to get my back against the building and someone took my arm.

"Can I help you?" a voice said.

Then I saw him.

"Can I help you?" he said again, and I looked at him as if he were speaking a foreign language.

"It's too late," I said incredulously, and it began as a low chuckle deep within me and grew louder and stronger with each breath.

The man looked around nervously to see if anyone was watching.

"It's too late." I laughed, and I heard my voice like a stranger's, formless and wild and terrible as the laughter rolled out of me.

The man, embarrassed, slipped away, and my body shook with the laughter as I slumped against the building, letting it take my weight. I didn't see the stares anymore. I didn't see the people anymore.

I leaned my head against the building and let the laughter come—until my eyes filled with tears, until my body trembled with gentle convulsions, until the sound caught in my throat, twisted into a gasp and then a sob. And then it began—a quiet weeping.

I tilted my head back and let the rain beat against my face, let it wash away the tears and the shame. I pushed myself off the building and walked across the parking lot, wiping at my eyes and nose with the back of my hand.

When I reached the car, the distant rumble of thunder brought memories of games and gods. They played to win, I thought. And they had won. Even the thought of their smug faces, smiling down victoriously at me, stirred no anger. Mortals always lost when matched against the gods. Thunder rolled across the sky and I looked up at the gods, and there it was— a small patch of summer blue in the storm-filled winter sky. Then it was gone, swallowed up by rolling clouds. "It's too late," I said bitterly. "It's just too late."

It didn't mean anything, that patch of blue. I once thought it did. I thought it did that day they pulled me from the ambulance, but I was so hurt and scared I would have believed anything. I was hurt and scared that day the coach kept running me up the middle time after time and it was there then, that patch of blue, and I was getting my brains kicked out. I would have kept getting 'em kicked out if I hadn't told the coach we were never going to make it up the middle. "Okay, run the ends," he had said.

Okay, run the ends. I laughed. It was simple then. It was a game then. If you couldn't run it up the middle, take it around the ends, and if they stopped you there, then throw the ball. Simple. But it wasn't a game now. There weren't any ends to run.

Or were there, I thought suddenly. If you can't do it one way—do it another. I wasn't trying to score a touchdown anymore, but I was trying to move from where I was to where I wanted to be, and I'd been trying to get there with a job. I'd been trying to run up the middle and they were knocking my brains out. I didn't have to have one of their jobs to get to where I wanted to be. There were other ways. I didn't have to work for someone else to have what I wanted. I could do it some other way. I could run the ends. By God, that patch of blue did mean something. It meant what it had always meant. It meant I could win.

I felt the blood begin to rise in my veins. My heart began to pound in my chest, and it wasn't anger this time. It was the same feeling I had had every time I pulled on a uniform or picked up a tennis racket or slipped on a pair of track shoes. It was the excitement of competition, the thrill of being in a game where you didn't have a chance and you knew you were going to win.

I'd run the ends and if they stopped me there I'd throw the ball and if that didn't work I'd try something else, but this game wasn't over, and that's what Cindy had failed to realize. You don't leave the field until the game is over, and you don't stand on the sidelines crying.

When I got home I went to my room and closed the door.

276

There had to be a way, if I could only think of it. I wasn't going on any more interviews—ever. There had to be something I could do on my own. Some kind of business. I would need capital for that, and that meant an interview where someone could say no. That was up the middle, and I was through getting my brains kicked out. But what could I do? How did I run the ends?

I sat down at my desk and noticed the two letters that had arrived with the morning mail—a lifetime ago. I picked them up and tossed them, unopened, into the wastebasket, picked up a pen and began to scribble nervously on the writing pad that lay on the desk. There had to be a way, I thought, and I printed the words in bold letters across the page.

I looked at those words for a long time. I lay down the pen and leaned back in the chair and sat staring at words printed across a page, and then I knew how I was going to run the ends. I tore off the top sheet of paper, wadded it up, and tossed it into the wastebasket.

I looked down at an empty white page and wondered if I could get it all down, all the anger, frustration, hope and loss of hope, all the work and pain and bitter disappointment.

I sat back in the chair and stared at a frighteningly blank sheet of paper. Stared at it until my life marched across that stark white plain like a colorful parade. They were all there— Rick and Mom, Stirewalt and Cindy, Harley, McKinnon, Bo, Jimmy Casteen and Curtis Rhinehardt, J.B., Althea . . . and Cory.

I reached for the pen, and thunder rumbled angrily across the sky like an admonition from the gods. I hoped they had placed their bets and I hoped they had wagered heavily, I thought with a smile, because I intended to win.